NEW MIRACLES
OF CHILDBIRTH

NEW MIRACLES
OF CHILDBIRTH

*What Modern Medicine Is Doing
to Make Childbearing
Safer and Easier*

by ELLIOTT H. McCLEARY

David McKay Company, Inc.

NEW YORK

Foreword

Today's expectant mother can approach childbirth with more confidence and peace of mind than was possible at any previous time.

She can do this primarily because of recent, rapid advances in the specialties of obstetrics, gynecology, and pediatrics. In the past decade we have seen tremendous gains in knowledge regarding all aspects of reproduction. Not only have effective hormonal and mechanical contraceptive methods been developed, but also improved methods of reversing infertility. We know far more about the growth and development and the maternal environment of the unborn baby. Management of pregnancy by the physician has become much more sophisticated, especially in the identification of certain pregnancies as high risk, in need of special attention. Finally, care of premature and critically ill newborns has evolved from the level of the old preemie nursery to the monitored ministrations of the newborn intensive-care unit.

Nonmedical forces have also figured importantly in making reproductive medicine one of today's most dynamic fields. There is public concern with the linked problems of overpopulation and the quality of human life. Changing public attitudes on abortion are reflected in and buttressed by new laws and judicial decisions. The medical and surgical care of pregnant women is affected significantly by the findings of investigations into the social aspects of disease and illness. And the advancement of the concept of women's liberation in all its connotations has had further impact on maternal and newborn management. Although not all of these forces have been entirely beneficial, there is no denying their influence.

The author of *New Miracles of Childbirth* has carried out extensive journalistic research on current developments in perinatal medicine, and has utilized acknowledged authorities as consultants to review his text. Not all physicians will agree with every statement in this book, nor indeed will all consumers and health-care providers; however, the author has highlighted most of the significant developments that will affect expectant parents in the years to come. The American College of Obstetricians and Gynecologists endorses all those efforts which will lead to ensuring comprehensive, high-quality obstetrical-gynecological care to every woman in our society—through solutions to the problems of maldistribution of health personnel and facilities, and the reduction of health-care costs by the more efficient use of current knowledge and services. Implementation of many of the advances reported in this book will contribute toward the achievement of that goal.

KEITH P. RUSSELL, M.D., F.A.C.O.G., F.A.C.S.
President, The American College of
Obstetricians and Gynecologists

Acknowledgments

This book was made possible only because of the great helpfulness and generosity of many uniquely qualified persons, including the following, who submitted to interviews, checked facts, gave advice, and contributed valuable reference materials. To them I am deeply indebted.

Dr. Karlis Adamsons, Dr. Gerald G. Anderson, Dr. Virginia Apgar, Beverly Aure, R.N., Dr. Kenneth E. Bell, Dr. Tom Brewer, Dr. Arnold Coran, Mrs. Frances Curry, Dorothy Davis, Dr. Maria Delivoria-Papadopoulas, Eunice K. M. Ernst, C.N.M., Dr. Roger Freeman, Dr. John B. Franklin, Mrs. Edwina Froehlich, Dr. Sprague Gardiner, Dr. John Grausz, Dr. Stanley N. Graven, Dr. J. Alex Haller, Jr., Dr. Stanley Harrison, Dr. Michael Hartigan, Dr. Joan E. Hodgman, Jay Hodin, Dr. Edward H. Hon, Albert W. Isenmen, Dr. L. Stanley James, Dr. Robert M. Kark, Charles W. Macenski, Dr. Robert Mendelsohn, Mike Michaelson, Dr. Niles Anne Newton, Dr. Erwin Nichols, Dr. Ben Peckham, Dr. Edward J. Quilligan, Dr. Robert E. Replogle, Dr. Arthur Salisbury, Dr. Barry Schifrin, Dr. Jack M. Schneider, Dr. Joseph O. Sherman, Dr. Leo Stern, Dr. Orvar Swenson, Dr. Philip L. White, Edith Wonnell, C.N.M., Dr. Sumner J. Yaffee, Dr. Frederick P. Zuspan.

The text of this book has been verified for accuracy, timeliness, and perspective by the following authorities:

Chapter I:	Charles W. Macenski Secretary, Committee on Maternal and Child Care American Medical Association
Chapters II, III:	Virginia Apgar, M.D., M.P.H. Vice President for Medical Affairs The National Foundation—March of Dimes
Chapter IV:	Philip L. White, Sc.D. Director, Department of Foods and Nutrition American Medical Association
Chapter V:	Karlis Adamsons, M.D., Ph.D. Professor, Department of Obstetrics and Gynecology Professor of Pharmacology Mount Sinai School of Medicine of the City University of New York
Chapter VI:	Sumner J. Yaffee, M.D. Professor of Pediatrics State University of New York at Buffalo
Chapters VII, VIII:	Barry Schifrin, M.D. Associate Professor of Obstetrics and Gynecology Harvard Medical School
Chapter IX:	L. Stanley James, M.D. Professor of Pediatrics

	College of Physicians and Surgeons
	of Columbia University; and Chairman, Committee on the Fetus and Newborn American Academy of Pediatrics
Chapter X:	A famous pediatric surgeon
Chapters XI, XII:	Jack M. Schneider, M.D. Associate Professor Department of Gynecology-Obstetrics and Pediatrics University of Wisconsin Center for Health Sciences Codirector, Wisconsin Perinatal Center, Madison
Chapter XII:	Stanley N. Graven, M.D. Professor of Pediatrics University of Wisconsin Center for Health Sciences Codirector, Wisconsin Perinatal Center, Madison
Chapter XIII:	Gerald G. Anderson, M.D. Chief of Obstetrics Yale Medical School
Chapter XIV:	Albert W. Isenman Administrator Office of Obstetric-Gynecologic Health Personnel American College of Obstetricians and Gynecologists
Chapter XV:	John B. Franklin, M.D. Chief of Staff Booth Maternity Center Philadelphia, Pennsylvania

Contents

NEW MIRACLES
OF CHILDBIRTH

CHAPTER

I

The Birth Frontier

We are beginning a new age in the ages old process of having a baby. It is a revolution that touches every aspect of maternal, unborn, and newborn life. And it has happened so suddenly that a woman who bore her last child five years ago may today return like Rip van Winkle to a far different world of childbirth.

This book is about that revolution and how it may affect the reader. It is a book not only for the mother-to-be but for her husband and her friends. It is for mothers of the future and for all persons who are intrigued by the excitement of a new frontier of medicine.

In every facet of our life today, this is the age of individual choice. And so it is in childbearing. Today's woman chooses when to conceive, and whether to proceed with her pregnancy. She has a choice of physicians using different methods, and she may have a choice of hospitals. She is torn between arguments for and against natural childbirth, breast-feeding, and the right of her mate to be at her side at the moment of birth. She is even urged by some to turn her back on doctors and hospitals and give birth with only her husband or lover attending, which can be dangerous.

This book can help her make wise choices.

The findings of science have placed new responsibilities on the shoulders of the mother-to-be. It is now known that the tranquilizers she takes even before she knows she is pregnant, the tobacco she smokes, the air she breathes, even the arguments she has with her husband may influence the development of her unborn baby. Every day she and sometimes her husband must make on-the-spot decisions affecting the course of her prenatal care.

A wise doctor to guide the pregnancy is more valuable than ever before; increased medical knowledge increases *his* options, tools, and makes his task more complex but also makes him more effective. But a wise patient is needed to make it a winning combination.

A woman no longer need fear pregnancy for her own sake, inconvenient or uncomfortable as it may be at times. Under good medical care, pregnancy today is not a threat to the life of the mother. Thanks to modern obstetrics and other specialties, that battle has been won. For every one hundred newborn deaths, there is only one maternal death. And when that death is investigated, it is found that the mother did not seek medical care or was out of reach of it. Or she died because of an illegal, botched abortion. Or she refused a therapeutic abortion. Or she did not have competent medical attention.

Last year in one populous Midwestern state, for example, there were only six maternal deaths associated with complications of pregnancy. I was assured by the director of the committee that investigates such deaths in that state that *every one* of the six fatalities could have been prevented by standard obstetrical care.

So when we speak in this book of high-risk pregnancies, in almost all cases we mean risk not to the mother but to the unborn. Rescuing him from death or lifelong damage is where the great problems and opportunities lie, where sometimes shocking conditions are still allowed to exist, where thousands of lives are still to be saved annually. Here and in the care of the newborn is the area of rapid change, ferment, discovery, and controversy we think of as the "birth frontier."

The birth frontier is only a few years old.

It was born with the advent of new knowledge about the fetus—knowledge, for example, that certain drugs taken by the mother could cross the placental barrier and alter the development of the baby.

It was born with new techniques, such as the sampling of amniotic fluid to detect abnormalities in the fetus or to judge its maturity.

It developed along with sophisticated medical equipment, such as the electronic fetal monitor. For the first time, doctors had a continuous record of the pulse of the unborn baby during labor and delivery. If trouble developed, they knew in time to prevent brain damage or stillbirth.

And the birth frontier was benefited by a radical new concept of nursing—intensive care. In complicated cases, "supernurses" apply their new knowledge minute by minute around the clock, aided by the complex equipment.

With the new knowledge has come a deeper psychological understanding of birth and the cementing of emotional bonds between husband and wife, parent and child. These bear on family stability and individual mental health when both seem threatened as never before.

We are speaking of this new frontier as if it is a present-day reality. And it is—at certain outposts at major medical centers across the nation, in most states, in most large cities and some smaller ones.

The birth frontier makes it possible for a woman pregnant *today* to cut her risk of stillbirth by one-third, her risk of infant mortality by half or more, and to reduce drastically the possibility that her child will suffer brain damage and subsequent learning or motor disorders. (These are figures quoted regularly by committees of the American College of Obstetricians and Gynecologists, the American Academy of Pediatrics, and the American Medical Association.)

But this is a period of transition. For most women, the birth frontier is five years off or more. There are not enough trained people, enough equipment, or enough public information so that everyone can benefit from it today. The frontier is unknown or imperfectly understood by a majority of mothers-to-be, nurses, doctors (even many doctors who deliver babies), and hospital administrators.

This book can help a mother-to-be seek out the outpost of the birth frontier nearest her (a few minutes' drive away for some readers, less than sixty for most). It can help her distinguish it from a unit that only appears to be a birth frontier outpost, such as a hospital that has renamed its maternity ward and its premature nursery without changing the substance of care delivered.

This book can help a woman determine whether her

doctor has access to the knowledge and facilities of the birth frontier. If he does not, it can help her select a doctor who does.

It can alert her to warning signs that her pregnancy may be high risk—and that she is in need of special attention not provided by routine care. It can help her discuss intelligently with her doctor whether her suspicions are groundless or whether she needs special resources—and how they can be provided for her.

The cheering news from the birth frontier is that high-risk pregnancies, if handled by the most modern means, often can be turned into low-risk cases. In fact, at certain advanced perinatal centers, including that of the University of Southern California, women categorized as high risk have been delivering with rates of fetal, maternal, and infant illness and mortality *below the national average* for all births.

The step from today into tomorrow's new world of obstetrical and newborn care will be a giant one. To glimpse that future and to tell about it here, the author has gone to the nation's best sources. He has interviewed the heads of the associations of America's obstetricians, pediatricians, and family physicians, the chairmen or secretaries of their committees on maternal and fetal and infant care, and a Congressional leader who is an obstetrician.

Across the land, he has interviewed leading obstetricians and pediatricians and chronicled their provocative, sometimes eloquent criticism of present-day practices that must and will be changed.

He has talked with mothers and fathers of healthy, normal, and vigorous babies who have been saved from certain death, mental retardation, or lifelong invalidism by modern miracles of the birth frontier.

In Boston's Beth Israel Hospital, he has shared a

young mother's excitement as an ultrasonic wand traced upon a screen the outlines of her unborn baby.

At Children's Memorial Hospital in Chicago, masked and gowned, he has stood at the elbow of a surgeon repairing an intestinal birth defect that would have killed the tiny newborn patient in a few days.

In Salt Lake City, he has traveled by ambulance with a doctor-nurse rescue team and a three-pound patient being rushed to the Intermountain Newborn Intensive Care Center at the University of Utah.

At the leading outposts of the birth frontier—including centers affiliated with the universities of Harvard, Columbia, Yale, Chicago, Wisconsin, Northwestern, Utah, and Southern California—he has observed at firsthand the drama of instrumented babies under plastic bubbles kept alive and restored to health by space-age medicine.

Everywhere, in conversations with leaders of the birth frontier, he has sensed an impatience with the status quo, a desire for greater public awareness of what could be done for mothers-to-be and their babies, an almost crusading zeal to change the system.

The vision of tomorrow's world of childbirth varies to some extent from one leader to another. But most agree upon the general outlines. All features of the new look are possible with the technology we have today. Although there may be no one place where all of these innovations are now in effect, all are in operation or are being developed at one place or another.

These changes can and will come, but, it was emphasized to me repeatedly, not nearly so fast as they should, unless an informed consumer public backs up medical and scientific leadership.

•Probably the most basic and fundamental advance

will be the interposition of a new layer of skilled personnel to assist in medical care, both in the physician's office and in the hospital. These doctors' helpers will record patient histories, conduct some examinations, follow up and follow through with patients to give them more time and attention than heretofore. In the hospital they will be trained to read electronic fetal monitoring systems and alert the doctor to dangerous patterns; they will assist in or perform deliveries; they will keep in touch with the patient after she returns home.

•A computer console may be used to record the patient's history. Closed-loop movies will help educate patients about diet, exercise, and special routines in a viewing room at the doctor's office. The doctor will "prescribe" reels 16, 24, 37, and 76, say, for a patient with four different health problems; such films are now in regular use in certain doctors' offices across the country, and are readily available to any doctor who wants to subscribe to the service.

•Computers will assist in patient diagnosis and may systematically remind doctors of necessary measures. A central monitoring agency keeping track of all pregnancies in a region could inform doctors of generally indicated procedures at appropriate times. (Still, the individual physician's knowledge of his patient and clinical judgment will remain the mother's best protection.)

•Each city, depending on its size, will contain only one or two hospitals with maternity services. A city the size of Washington, D.C., for instance, will have two services, each serving a half of the city and adjacent suburban regions. Each hospital maternity service will have attached to it a high-risk clinic for obstetrical complications from conception onward. Next door to the maternity department in the hospital will be a newborn intensive-care unit for critically ill or premature babies, to save them by means of special equipment, constant attention, and superskilled nursing and medical care. On call will be a full range of specialists—from doctors of internal medicine especially expert in kidney trouble (a frequent complicating factor in pregnancies) to surgeons skilled in repairing birth defects—shortly after birth. Associated laboratories will provide an increasingly sophisticated array of services to protect mothers-to-be, the unborn, and newborns.

"Perinatal center" is the term for this total complex (which is usually part of a much larger medical center and affiliated with a medical school). Obviously, not every town of 25,000 or even 100,000 will have the resources for a full-fledged center; these smaller communities will send maternity cases to nearby centers or establish limited facilities linked with the region's perinatal center.

•All births will be monitored electronically from the inception of labor. Fetal monitors will also probably be used in certain instances to answer questions about the baby's condition weeks before birth. Despite the addition of expensive, complex scientific equipment, mothers will get more personal attention, not less.

•The costs of having a baby will rise. Technology and additional personnel are expensive—and yet a bargain in the long run, considering the stakes.

•In the new world of childbirth, there will be a unified effort to care for and protect the patient— more cooperation and referral among doctors and hospitals, shared use of laboratory facilities; this will eliminate the grossly wasteful competition now present among hospitals that duplicate facilities in the same region, each hoping to boast the best and the most. As there is currently in Arizona, Wisconsin, and Indiana, there will be provisions for a "hot line" to regional perinatal centers so that any doctor in a region at any time of the day or night can get needed consultation in a complicated obstetrical case, without delay or embarrassment.

•As there is now in Wisconsin and several nearby Midwestern states, there will be regional perinatal associations composed of doctors, nurses (and eventually representatives of the public) to promote the best possible prenatal, birth, and postnatal care to all of the patients in each region. In such a body, nurses and concerned lay persons will share leadership with physicians.

•Political action groups will be formed to urge hospital trustees to close small, obsolescent maternity services, to get funds for perinatal centers from public bodies, and to persuade insurance companies and health-care organizations to broaden financial coverage of intensive perinatal care. There will be pressure —hopefully initiated by concerned physicians—to insist on refresher courses and periodic recertifying examinations for all doctors and specialized allied health professionals who deliver babies or assist in the process. Expectant mothers will be more strongly encouraged to take advantage of the available services, which many today do not.

In the new world of childbirth, newborn mortality will be lowered to what now seems an irreducible level of four per thousand live births. Some regions may reach this figure, which is one-fourth the best state rates of 1965, within a year.

And miracles such as the following will happen every day somewhere in America. (All are *presently* possible.)

Up to three out of four babies faced with mental retardation will be saved from it by improved obstetrics.

Ten babies per day will be prevented from certain disastrous birth defects because their mothers refrained from eating potatoes (which now affect up to one in one thousand births in the United States, one in one hundred in potato-eating Ireland).

Certain infant victims of a rare birth defect, combined immune deficiency, will spend the first months of their lives untouched by human hands in plastic isolation chambers where germs cannot reach them. Eventually, as happened with twin boys so protected for three years in Ulm, Germany, their bodies' immunity systems will slowly mature so they can live normally. Or bone-marrow transplants may enable their bodies to develop immunity.

A mother-to-be will be able to discover the sex of her unborn child in the fourth month of pregnancy, through the simple testing of a drop of her saliva. The procedure will be useful in predicting sex-linked birth defects (such as hemophilia, which affects only boys).

The number of Rh babies, half of whom now die, will continue to decline steadily in number until the disease becomes in fact a rarity; their condition can even now be prevented. Better care for those that are born will reduce mortality.

"Bad boys" and "slow learners" in schools will decrease because of better methods of delivering babies and caring for newborns, which will reduce subtle brain damage that affects personality, motor control, and learning ability.

More babies will be delivered with little or no use

of anesthetics, through such techniques as prepared childbirth, natural childbirth, and hypnosis. There will be further experiments in various parts of the United States with electroanesthesia and acupuncture to relieve labor pain. (In Chicago, in March 1973, newspaper reporter Linda Lee Landis gave birth under acupuncture anesthesia administered by Wei-Chi Liu, M.D.)

Nine out of ten babies afflicted with hyaline membrane disease will recover, thanks to new techniques. The condition, which killed the infant son of President and Mrs. Kennedy, has traditionally accounted for more than 25,000 infant deaths a year.

More births in the near tomorrow will take place in a setting of blinking lights, green glowing cathode-ray screens, dials and wires and tubes. For patients who do not know what to expect, the effect at first may be frightening.

But each mother-to-be will be the object of more human concern and psychological understanding. More, not fewer people will be taking care of her. They will know what they are doing, and will be assisted by machines keeping a moment-by-moment watch on the true condition of her and her unborn baby. All of the resources of modern obstetrics will be at their ready command for her protection.

Knowing this, a woman can take comfort. In every way, she and her baby are far safer than were she and her own mother at her own birth a short generation before.

These years, of all times in the history of giving birth, are and will be the very best time to have a baby!

CHAPTER

II

Prenatal Care: Earlier and Earlier

It happens every day at most big hospitals:

A frightened pregnant girl enters, informs Admissions that she is in the throes of labor, and is rushed to the maternity ward.

This is the first time during her pregnancy that she has seen a doctor. And it is too late for most of his skills in preventing mishaps to her or her baby.

The grim odds in such cases negatively indicate the value of prenatal care. In Baltimore, for example, just prior to 1960, a study by A. L. Haskins revealed that mothers under sixteen years old who received no prenatal care lost one infant for each eleven delivered. If they received such care, infant mortality was cut by two-thirds.

As late as 1972, The National Foundation—March of Dimes stated that "Municipal hospitals report that between one-third and one-half of women in labor have had little or no medical care prior to hospitalization."

Women who do not get prenatal care today are usually the poor and little educated. The average American woman is convinced of the value of medical help during pregnancy.

Before She Knows. Increasingly, however, the American woman will be urged by experts to protect her offspring during the moments, days, and weeks just after conception, when she may not even know she's pregnant. "This is *the* important time for preventing abnormalities in the fetus," I was told by the world-renowned Dr. Virginia Apgar, medical director of The National Foundation—March of Dimes. Thus, until contraception becomes 100 percent perfect, a sexually active woman must guard against possible fetal damage throughout her fertile years.

Estimates of the critical period, says Dr. Apgar, range from sixty days after conception, by University of California at Davis geneticist Alexander Barry, down to forty days, by geneticist James G. Wilson of the University of Cincinnati. It is generally accepted that the fetal nervous system forms during days fifteen to twenty-five after conception, the limbs in days twenty-four to thirty-six, the heart in days twenty-eight to forty-five, fingers and toes during days thirty-six to forty-two, ears and nose in days twenty-nine to forty-five. Thus an insult to the fetus, such as a powerful drug taken by his mother, may at thirty days' development cause foreshortened limbs, at forty days, blindness.

"So," says Dr. Apgar, "at the end of two months, maybe before the mother has seen a doctor to confirm her pregnancy, you can forget about abnormal development."

Exceptions, she notes, are formation of enzymes "about which we know practically nothing" and myelin and bone formation.

One of the most important advances in obstetrics,

believes Dr. Apgar, will be a test to detect pregnancy before implantation in the womb of the fertilized egg. The best in use today don't reveal pregnancy until almost three weeks after conception—halfway through the critical period of organ development.

Thus, even before she misses her menstrual period, an unaware mother may subject her fetus to possibly dangerous abdominal X rays, migraine medicine, tranquilizers, insecticide spray—to any of a vast array of everyday drugs and chemicals suspected of causing birth defects. To guard against this danger, Danish radiologist Kirsten Nøkkentved recommends that abdominal or pelvic X rays in fertile women be restricted whenever possible to the first two weeks after the last period.

In the absence of an early test for pregnancy, many women in the past have panicked upon missing a period and submitted to an illegal and unnecessary abortion procedure. Worry about a nonexistent pregnancy has sent many a girl into an emotional tailspin.

Until recently, a pregnancy test meant the sending of a urine sample away to a laboratory, and days of delay. Physicians now can apply a dot of the patient's urine to a card, wait two minutes, and read the verdict under a microscope. Manufacturers of the Prognosticon Dri-Dot, who also make a more accurate two-hour office test, recommend routine use for *all* fertile women before an X ray, an immunization, or any procedure that might harm a fetus.

The latter tests eliminate laboratory delay, but like the older methods they depend upon detection of a hormone, human chorionic gonadotrophin (HCG) produced by the new placenta beginning two weeks after implantation of the fertilized egg in the uterus. A Swedish test under study, which detects a different hormone, is reported to reveal pregnancy eight days after implantation.

In the Netherlands, women can buy a self-test pregnancy kit called the Predictor, said to give an answer in twenty seconds, with 98-percent accuracy. A similar test kit sold in England is called Twentisec. And, suggests Dr. Morris Fishbein, warning of the need for regulation, it is likely that such tests will soon be appearing in the United States. There is a danger that these will be distributed by illegal or unethical abortion clinics, or even sold in connection with do-it-yourself abortion kits. (Recently the American Medical Association learned of a $2 mail-order self-abortion device designed to hook up to and be powered by the patient's home vacuum cleaner.)

Women who do not wish to be pregnant will soon be able to prevent pregnancy with a morning-after pill taken within seventy-two hours after intercourse. In experimental use now at the University of Wisconsin and other centers around the world, it is based upon a synthetic version of prostaglandin, which causes strong contraction of smooth muscle and is found in nature in human semen and menstrual fluid.

"Birth control will presently become a nonproblem," says Dr. Eric G. Saint, medical dean at the University of Queensland, Australia, "because of the use of prostaglandins. It is possible that the world population problem will simply disappear." (Two prostaglandins have been cleared for use by physicians in selected clinics and hospitals in the United Kingdom; general U.S. use will probably not be allowed before 1975.)

Those who fail to take their morning-after pills in time have a new recourse. It is a revolutionary form of pregnancy test that promises to eliminate the need for most abortions with their resulting mental anguish, physical risk, and expense. Known as "menstrual regulation," it can be done in a minute or two in a doctor's office, and is now being pioneered by physicians across the country.

A woman who fears she is pregnant and wishes to be "regulated" visits her physician within two weeks after her missed period. Without medication, he inserts through her undilated cervix a flexible plastic tube attached to a special syringe. The syringe then quickly sucks out the menstrual lining, and with it, if present, the fertilized egg. Since in practice no determination of pregnancy is made, menstrual regulation is not likely to provoke the guilt that may be caused by an abortion. And the cost is around $30 rather than the $150 or more of an abortion.

Do-it-yourself menstrual regulation has been initiated by several vocal feminist groups which distribute a menstrual extraction device similar to that used by physicians. But, according to Dr. Alan Guttmacher, Director of the Planned Parenthood Federation, "anybody who attempts to do it herself should know that she is courting disaster."

Abortions and even menstrual regulation represent emergency action for an initial failure—conception control. The perfect contraceptive still remains to be invented.

One disadvantage of oral contraceptive pills, according to Dr. S. B. Effer of McMaster University, Hamilton, Ontario, Canada, could be a residual effect that for a time after use might possibly pose a danger to a fetus. He advises women not to become pregnant immediately after they stop using birth-control pills, or just after removal of an intrauterine device (IUD).

Abortions may also pose a danger to future children by causing some to be born prematurely, it was indicated by surveys disclosed at the Sixth World Congress of Gynecology and Obstetrics in 1970. In seven East European countries where abortion has been legal since the mid-fifties, the proportion of premature births increases with the frequency of abortion. Thus, in Hungary, according to 1968 figures, the rate of premature births among women who had no induced abortion was 10 percent; with one, 14 percent; with two, 18 percent, and with three or more, 24 percent. Similar findings have been reported from Japan.

One apparently hazard-free "natural" method of birth control recently resulted in a Papal Knighthood bestowed by Pope Paul on its chief developer, Dr. John J. Billings, M.D., of Melbourne University, Melbourne, Australia. The simple technique, tested on more than one thousand women in Melbourne, depends upon avoiding intercourse in the days following ovulation, which is recognized by discharge for four or five days of clear, slippery mucus from the cervix. During "safe" periods the mucus is cloudy and tacky.

Many women in the experiment are now successfully instructing others in use of the technique, according to Dr. Billings, including five hundred women in the South Pacific kingdom of Tonga and even fifty blind women in Melbourne. The method is also being promoted in Latin America.

One important drawback, also shared by the Church-approved but unreliable rhythm method, has been hinted at by Dr. Billings:

"Many husbands," he has said, "claim that they are able to tell when their wives are ovulating by their increased energy and flirtatious behavior."

Yet this is the time, when the woman's sexual appetite is at its height, that the mucous method keeps mates apart.

An important pre-prenatal step for the one woman

in seven who has Rh-negative blood, to protect future children against Rh disease, must be taken within seventy-two hours after a miscarriage or abortion, as well as after birth of an Rh-positive baby. Injection of Rh immunoglobulin (Rho-gam is a trade name) will prevent her immunity system from producing antibodies against red blood cells from her baby which at delivery entered her bloodstream. If she does not get the injection, she may develop antibodies that during her next pregnancy will cross the placenta into the baby's bloodstream, and destroy the child's Rh-positive blood cells.

Until introduction of Rh isoimmunization in 1968–1969, one U.S. baby in two hundred was affected; over half died in the womb or shortly after birth. And many of those who lived were born severely ill. Not even intrauterine transfusions, the most famous obstetric technique of the 1960s, nor transfusions and treatment immediately after birth, could save all.

Isoimmunization, the immunoglobulin technique, promises virtually to wipe out Rh disease complications in a single generation. But it will happen only if proper steps are taken after abortions and miscarriages as well as births.

Before Pregnancy. Many doctors now stress to future mothers the need for good prenatal care before pregnancy: proper diet, weight control, enough exercise and sleep in the months before pregnancy, so the fetus from its beginning will have the best possible home.

The concept is known as "preconceptional care."

Writing in *Hospital Medicine*, Robert E. L. Nesbitt, Jr., M.D., and Richard H. Aubry, M.D., of the State University of New York Upstate Medical Center in Syracuse argue for even earlier attention.

They recommend a detailed medical history, laboratory tests, and a thorough physical examination just before marriage when the prospective bride appears for the compulsory blood test for syphillis.

Nesbitt and Aubry have found genital tract problems in 10 percent of their examined brides-to-be, in addition to other disorders which may affect pregnancy, such as diabetes. "This preventative approach," they say, "may have far greater influence in assuring successful gestation than energetic treatment during pregnancy."

Immunization is another important form of preconceptional care. Prospective brides in Illinois must now give proof that they have been tested for immunity to rubella (German measles) which can cause severe damage to a fetus during the first three months of pregnancy. The law does not force her to become immunized, explains Fred Uhlig of the Illinois Department of Public Health. In fact, he explains, the shot ideally should not be administered less than six months before a pregnancy begins, because it gives the woman a mild case of the disease, which could affect her unborn child (persistence of rubella vaccine-like virus has been noted for as long as sixty-nine days after a shot by the national Center for Disease Control). If she is already pregnant at the time of marriage, or is planning to conceive soon, her doctor is likely to suggest that she get a shot immediately after having her first child.

Never again, it appears, will the unborn babies of the nation suffer a rubella assault like the epidemic of 1964–1965, which caused 50,000 to die in the womb or to be born with severe defects including deafness, blindness, and mental retardation. Mass vaccinations of all children under twelve are expected to eliminate the rubella menace.

A combination measles-mumps-rubella vaccine now in use may eliminate additional hazards to future fetuses. Mumps, for example, has been suspected of causing a fetal heart disease affecting one birth in 10,-000. Dr. Guy McKhann of Johns Hopkins University Medical School has caused the birth defect hydrocephalus (water on the brain, causing the head to swell) in fetal hamsters by injecting their mothers with mumps virus. Infection caused by various viruses, suggests McKhann, could block off fetal drainage ducts to cause the condition, once thought to be inherited.

America's future mothers face a growing hazard of possible sterility from what has become the second-most-frequent communicable disease in the United States, trailing only the common cold: gonorrhea.

"Gonorrhea is truly epidemic," according to Dr. J. Donald Miller of the national Center for Disease Control. He estimates that there are about 2.5 million cases each year in the United States.

Some estimates are even higher. *Emergency Medicine* magazine reports that "Tests for gonorrhea . . . have shown that about *one in ten* girls between the ages of 15 and 25 has gonorrhea and doesn't know it. By the time they do become aware of it, it is a serious complication that could render them sterile or subject to ectopic pregnancy, which requires immediate surgical intervention, or simply leaves them gynecological cripples."

In 1972, the Federal Government began a campaign to urge physicians to include a gonorrhea test, along with the usual Pap smear, in the periodic pelvic examination of every fertile American woman. And at about the same time, a simplified office screening test, Clinicult, was introduced.

Sexually active men and boys were urged by public

health and medical spokesmen not to desist, but to protect against VD's spread by returning to use of the condom, abandoned with the advent of the Pill.

At the second International Venereal Disease Symposium, Dr. William M. Edwards announced that Progonasyl, a contraceptive vaginal preparation, is apparently successful in protecting women against VD. Edwards, chief of Preventive Medical Services of the State of Nevada, proved the drug in an unusual controlled setting—with the cooperation of the 324 inmates of Nevada's forty legal houses of prostitution. (The only side effect: drying of the vagina in some women who perform multiple sex acts on the same day.)

As gonorrhea becomes more resistant to penicillin, and to other antibiotics, new methods of treatment are sought. Among the remedies is Spectinomycin, which in final tests by the Center for Disease Control has proved to have a 95-percent cure rate with administration of only one shot.

Vaccines seem to promise the final answer for VD.

A syphilis vaccine is being sought by several investigators in this country, and an experimental vaccine in rabbits has been tested in Poland. But most scientists are not optimistic about the chances of a human vaccine soon.

A gonorrhea vaccine has already been developed in Canada, and under Canadian government auspices is undergoing a large-scale clinical test among the students of Makerere University, Uganda. Up to two thousand volunteers from the university community, which has a high rate of venereal disease, were expected to participate. And strong indications of the effectiveness of the vaccine were expected to show at the end of the trial's first year of testing.

Mating roulette. Increasingly, young people will become aware of a fact long known to livestock breeders: good prenatal care includes picking a genetically appropriate mate.

Many common birth defects and genetic diseases could be avoided completely, before marriage, by genetic counseling.

Thus, if a girl carrying a gene for cystic fibrosis marries a boy who also has the gene, their chances of producing a CF child are one in four—each time a child is born. If neither marries a carrier, the odds are overwhelming that none of their children will be CF-afflicted.

Similarly, sex-linked inherited conditions like hemophilia and color blindness—affecting only males —afflict 50 percent of the sons born to couples in which both mates carry the gene.

Much diabetes is thought to be caused by a genetic defect; so are many other diseases appearing first in youth or middle age.

A defective gene making the bearer prone to emphysema affects 5 percent of the U.S. population—10 percent of all those of northern European ancestry. Most emphysema victims have it.

Some two thousand genetic defects in humans have been identified.

All in all, estimates Stanford University's Joshua Lederberg, Nobel Prize-winning biologist, "at least 25 percent of all hospital beds and of all institutional places for the handicapped in this country are occupied by persons suffering from some sort of genetic disease."

But how soon, if ever, will genetic considerations enter into human mate selection? Will the day come when a boy and girl trade genetic histories at the time that they exchange class rings?

It seems obvious that public interest in and use of genetic counseling will continue to grow at a faster rate than the increase in the number of genetic counselors.

There are now more than 150 genetic counseling services in the nation, most of them located in large medical centers and funded largely by research grants. Under present conditions the process of genetic analysis is laborious and would be prohibitively expensive if it were not for the support of research funds, including those of the Federal Government and The National Foundation—March of Dimes.

If even a fraction of brides and grooms presented themselves for genetic analysis, the counselors would be swamped. Nor could they be too definite in many of their predictions in these early stages of a burgeoning science. For many of the causes of genetic defects are complex and interrelated, still to be fathomed.

Young people contemplating marriage today are advised to seek genetic counseling if any brother, sister, or parent has a serious condition caused by a genetic disease such as muscular dystrophy, Huntington's chorea, or hemophilia.

Genetic counseling for all should begin with the physician who gives the premarital examination, believes Dr. Leon Peris of Jefferson Medical College in Philadelphia. Taking a thorough family history (together, suggests Dr. Apgar, with blood, urine, and tissue samples) from both future mates may reveal dangers ahead, a procedure that seems more sensible and merciful than the current practice in which aid is not sought until after the birth of a deformed child. In some cases a couple may opt for sterilization and adoption instead of childbearing. Actually, says Dr. Peris, "In the vast majority of situations, the risk factors are so low that we can reassure the patient."

Genetic screening programs seem to be a wave of the future.

In the Washington, D.C.–Baltimore, Maryland, area, blood samples from 60,000 couples have been taken to detect carriers of Tay-Sachs disease, which causes loss of coordination, seizures, blindness, and death usually by the age of five. (Primarily, it is found among descendants of Ashkenazic Jews, who originally lived in a small area near the Russian-Polish border.)

Dr. Michael M. Kaback, director of the pilot program, predicts that similar programs will be used to discover carriers of other diseases caused by recessive genes. He stipulates three requirements:

"The disease must occur in a defined population group, there must be a simple, accurate, and inexpensive carrier detection test, and it must be possible to detect the disease early in pregnancy" (so an affected fetus can be aborted).

All blacks in America are potential candidates to be tested for sickle-cell anemia, the gene for which is carried by 8 to 10 percent of this population. One black child in four hundred is born with the condition, which cannot be detected in amniotic fluid (in the future, fetal blood samples may be taken).

Mass screening has become practical with development of a simple ten-minute screening test, easily learned by volunteer technologists, that costs only five cents per sample. The test, announced in late 1971, can distinguish between persons carrying the sickle-cell anemia trait and those suffering from the disease. It also can detect five other blood disorders.

If administered to all young blacks before parenthood, the test would enable a sickle-cell carrier to avoid marrying another—and thus avoid the possibility of children afflicted with the disease.

Brave New World. In the future, believe many researchers, it will be possible to cure such genetic defects as sickle-cell anemia and Tay-Sachs disease by genetic engineering either in young adults, in the fetus, or even before conception. A harmless virus carrying a corrective gene will be allowed to invade the subject cells and fuse with them, adding the desired genetic detail.

Thus, experiments at the National Institutes of Health have shown that a bacterial virus known as a lambda phage will correct galactosemia. This is a genetic condition caused by a deficiency of enzymes required to metabolize the sugar galactose; it can result in brain damage and eye cataracts. In laboratory experiments the carrier virus transferred the healthy gene that prevents galactosemia to cells taken from a child afflicted with the disease.

Vasken Aposhia at the University of Maryland is seeking to find the gene or genes which control the body's production of insulin, which controls diabetes. If he does so, and is able to synthesize these genes, he would employ a virus to pick up the genetic information and transfer it to human body cells.

Aposhia is considering injection of the genetic information into diabetic children. But it may become possible to treat a child soon after his conception—either inside or outside the womb. It would also be possible to inspect the developing blastocyst—the cluster of cells developing from the fertilized human egg—and reject a genetically or chromosomally defective specimen, such as an incipient Mongoloid child.

The birth of the first test-tube baby—the first human in history conceived outside a human body—quite possibly will have occurred by the time this book is published.

The techniques have already been developed and proved in veterinary medicine.

In Australia, veterinary scientists working with sheep inject a prize ewe with a chemical that causes her to hyperovulate—to produce twenty-nine or thirty eggs ripening all at once. They take them out, fertilize them with choice sperm (selected either for superior meat or wool qualities) and then implant these genetically superior embryos into the wombs of twenty-nine ordinary sheep.

The same technique is now being employed with cattle on the 1346-acre ranch of James E. Dula, Jr., near Marietta, Oklahoma. More than a dozen healthy Hereford calves have been produced from eggs fertilized in the laboratory and implanted in foster mothers, in a breeding experiment conducted by veterinarian Dr. Duane C. Kraemer (who is also engaged in research into the reproductive physiology of primates).

News of the first successful human test-tube babies, it appears at this writing, will come from Oxford, England, and the Cambridge University physiology laboratories of Dr. Robert G. Edwards. Or it may originate from Oldham General Hospital near Manchester, where Edwards' babies are to be delivered.

Happily cooperating with Edwards are some fifty women, most of them in their middle thirties, who cannot produce children in the usual way because their Fallopian tubes are blocked. The eggs their ovaries produce heretofore had not been able to reach the uterus, nor could sperm from their husbands fertilize the eggs.

At the time each volunteer ovulates, Dr. Edwards inserts through her navel a thin, lighted, metal probe known as a laparoscope, which retrieves a ripe ovum from the egg sac. In a laboratory dish he exposes the captured ovum to sperm collected from the woman's husband, then for days harbors the fertilized egg in an incubator until its cells have multiplied many times. Finally, with a laparoscope, he implants the fertilized egg, now known as a blastocyst, into the uterine wall of the mother. Pregnancy then proceeds in the usual manner, with normal birth nine months later.

The Future. The Oxford trials suggest an intriguing array of possibilities in pre-prenatal medicine:

In the future, a couple with defective genes may ask a genetic laboratory to perform an artificial conception of their sperm and ovum. The developing blastocyst could be inspected for genetic defects before implantation; or if a gene is missing, it could be added using a gene-carrying virus.

In the Edwards experiments, the developing embryos are intensively studied under a microscope to identify damage caused by handling, and also to spot certain original genetic defects, including those leading to Mongolism.

Embryo implantation in the next few years could mean fertility for one-fourth of all sterile women— those unable to bear children because of blocked or missing Fallopian tubes.

It could mean motherhood for women with defective genes or the inability to produce ova of their own, by means of donated eggs, fertilized by their husbands' semen, implanted in their wombs. Some may become pregnant because of an ovary transplant, as happened in 1972 to a young Argentine woman operated upon by Dr. Raul Blanco in Buenos Aires.

Such measures will seem increasingly attractive to childless couples as improved contraception and rising abortions shut off the flow of unwanted children —the chief source of adoptions today. The woman who wishes to adopt will do so, but at an earlier stage. She, rather than a teen-ager who has made a "mistake," will happily undergo gestation and delivery of the child she will rear.

A woman who has undergone a hysterectomy could even become a mother—provided she could find another woman willing to bear her child.

Legal and ethical considerations may, in some countries, delay such innovations. But the technical means to perform them are at hand.

CHAPTER

III

On the Trail of Teratogens: The Case of the Blighted Potato

Of all the mysteries solved by Sherlock Holmes, perhaps none was as strange and baffling. Nor had Holmes ever pursued a villain as vicious as the one tracked across the globe by James H. Renwick, a scientific detective of modern-day London.

Piecing together a host of clues from many sources, Renwick has indicted with damning evidence what seems an important crippler and killer of unborn babies—something we have all eaten from time to time: the ordinary white potato, which manufactures a powerful antifungus chemical when it is affected by a common blight.

"The case of the blighted potato" promises to go down in medical history as the most celebrated story of a teratogen since the thalidomide disaster. A teratogen is an agent or factor producing a physical defect in a developing embryo. Some teratogens are mutagens as well; a mutagen causes genetic damage that is transmitted to succeeding generations. And in the past few years, since the thalidomide disaster, the search for teratogens has broadened to place under suspicion a host of common substances that have caused abnormalities in animal fetuses.

For the expectant mother, the subject of teratogens can be frightening. But she should be encouraged that possible fetus-harming agents are at last being identified so that they can be avoided and removed from the environment.

"Teratogens were always there," the March of Dimes' Dr. Virginia Apgar pointed out to me. "We are just now recognizing them."

Furthermore, she adds, the fact that a tranquilizer or food additive causes defects in animals does not necessarily mean it will harm humans.

"It's a general principle that the defect has to be observed in the species you're studying. Thus, thalidomide in humans only—and some baboons and chimpanzees—caused shortness of the limbs and abnormalities of the external ears and diaphragm. But rabbits got twisted bones and rats got cleft palate, which didn't happen at all with human beings."

Most hopeful of all is the present belief of geneticists, as stated by The National Foundation—March of Dimes, that only 20 percent of birth abnormalities are inherited.

Another 20 percent are solely environmentally caused, by such things as X rays or an illness afflicting the mother, such as rubella.

"Rubella is in a class by itself," says Dr. Apgar, "because its damage is done primarily through the route of infection. Most rubella defects in the 1964–1965 epidemic were caused directly by disease of the fetus—infection, for example, of a perfectly normal lens of the eye and inner ear. There was nothing the matter with the genes of the fetus; it simply caught the disease from its mother. Even then, only half of the babies became sick when their mothers contracted rubella during pregnancy."

Like rubella, much or all of environmental causes of damage can be avoided once they are identified. Conceivably so can much or all of the remaining 60 percent of malformations, which require not only an offending agent but a hereditary susceptibility to it. An example may be cleft palate, which is more likely to run in certain family strains, but does not do so according to known laws of genetics. Possibly an outside chemical agent is needed to induce the defect in a susceptible fetus.

All of which indicates that birth defects prevention is in its early days of exploration, at about the same stage that geography was in when sailors were sighting sea serpents and Columbus discovered the New World but thought he'd landed in India. And the saga of James H. Renwick and his search for the potato teratogen will be only one of many such ventures to succeed in the years just ahead.

Renwick, a geneticist at the London School of Hygiene and Tropical Medicine, announced his theory in 1972 that women who eat blighted potatoes during the first month of their pregnancy may, as a result, give birth to babies born with spina bifida and/or anencephaly.

The two defects occur at about the same rate, times, and places, in markedly parallel but differing incidences in different countries. Spina bifida, characterized by a cleft in the spinal column, can be severely crippling and frequently is fatal. Anencephaly invariably is fatal, for it prevents formation of the top of the head, including the brain.

Renwick, in an exhaustive search of agricultural and medical literature, correlated outbreaks of potato blight all over the world with subsequent epidemics of anencephaly and spina bifida.

He found the greatest incidence in the world of the birth defects to occur, appropriately, in Ireland. Not only do the people of Ireland eat a great quantity of potatoes, but the island's wet climate makes blight a perennial problem for potato growers. (It was this same blight, now prevalent around the world, that destroyed the Irish potato crop and caused the great potato famine of 1848.)

Similarly, potato blight is more prevalent in wetter eastern Canada than in the drier west—and the combined total of anencephaly and spina bifida falls correspondingly from the wet east—2.93 per thousand births in Quebec—to the drier west—1.03 in British Columbia. The same pattern is found in the United States; potatoes from dry Idaho are far safer than those from moist Maine.

Renwick found that southern Japanese, who eat few potatoes, have a low incidence of the two birth defects —.8 per thousand—and that the county in Norway with the severest potato blight also has the highest rate of mortality from spina bifida. He found that the lower occupational classes in England, who eat more potatoes (because they are cheap food) than the upper classes, have far more incidence of the two defects.

Discovering that a higher rate of defects occurred in large family units than in small, he placed the blame on the size of the batch prepared for a typical meal: the more cooked together, the greater the odds that one would contaminate the lot. And he used a seeming exception to prove the rule: first-born children are more susceptible to the defects because a large percentage are conceived prior to marriage, when the mother still lives at home with brothers, sisters, parents, and often grandparents.

Despite enough proof to convince a layman ten times over, Renwick modestly called his proposal a "hypothesis" pending the outcome of experiments under way with pregnant marmoset monkeys fed blighted potatoes. But he did suggest these precautions for potentially pregnant women:

•Discard any potato that has brownish or blackish bruises on the white meat, a condition easiest to spot at the time of peeling. *Do not* merely cut out the dark spot. It is not the spot that creates the poison believed to cause spina bifida, it is the potato itself that manufactures the suspect toxins phytuberin, rishitin, and lubimin—actually antibiotics designed to kill the potato blight fungus. Avoid such potatoes not only during the critical first month of "hidden pregnancy" but for the first four months—to rule out the possibility of any other kind of damage to the fetus. (Since many pregnancies are unexpected, even in these days of the Pill and IUD, it is really safest to observe all of the precautions listed here throughout the childbearing years.)

•A woman who may be pregnant can cut her odds of being exposed to a blighted potato by boiling her own spuds in a small pan separately from those of the rest of the household.

•A woman who has already borne a child affected with spina bifida or anencephaly is at a 5-percent risk of having another; there seems to be a hereditary susceptibility. She can reduce her risk by reducing her exposure to potatoes.

•A final possibility discussed by Renwick is that a pregnant woman may absorb the toxin not through eating, but simply by breathing the vapor emitted by boiling potatoes. This, then, is to be avoided.

•Not mentioned by Renwick but following from his suggestions: Any woman who may be pregnant should avoid eating any potatoes she herself has not prepared—as at a restaurant or a friend's house.

•Instant dehydrated potatoes are "probably" free of the blight, Renwick has told reporters.

How many more birth defects are caused by unsuspected everyday substances like the common potato? And what of the new chemicals constantly being introduced into our environment?

Dr. Charles U. Lowe, scientific director of the National Institute of Child Health and Human Development warns, "We live in cities smothered in smog, rear children within the shadow of industrial behemoths that belch forth noxious fumes, and eat food that is contaminated by defoliants, pesticides, estrogens, androgens, and antimicrobial agents. The convenience food industry has grown like a malignant sore, including in the package preservatives, emulsifiers, antioxidants, coloring agents, and flavoring."

Dr. Sydney S. Gellis, of Tufts University School of Medicine, urges that "Nothing whatsoever of unknown toxicity should be introduced into the environment, either as pesticide, herbicide, defoliant, insect repellent or food additive. The teratogenic [defect-causing] effect is the vital key. Any agent found to be toxic or teratogenic in test animals should be excluded from public use."

A Food and Drug Administration program to test and study all food additives for possible fetal damage began in 1972. But that alone, as Dr. Apgar has pointed out, is not enough.

"There is no valid and conservative basis for predicting relative sensitivities to chemicals between humans and animals," agrees Dr. Samuel S. Epstein, professor of pharmacology at Case Western Reserve University School of Medicine. He points out that Meclizine, an antihistamine drug used for treating morning sickness, causes birth defects in rats but not in humans who have been studied. On the other hand, "humans are sixty times more sensitive to thalidomide than mice, one hundred times more sensitive than rats, two hundred times more sensitive than dogs, and seven hundred times more sensitive than hamsters."

National health leaders have campaigned for an "early warning system" that would collect and retrieve data on defects in newborns and especially in aborted fetuses, and try quickly to identify causes of upswings or clusters of birth defects.

"Some of us have been pleading for a congenital malformations surveillance program for nearly a decade," Dr. Robert L. Brent of Jefferson Medical College told the Teratology Society in 1970. "We are still pleading. If German physicians had had the simplest birth-defects screening program back in 1961, they would have detected thalidomide damage after twenty-five babies, not five thousand."

"The feasibility of computerized monitoring of births nationwide," announced The National Foundation—March of Dimes in 1972, "is being explored to develop an early warning system of 'epidemics' of certain birth defects which may be related to environmental agents."

Vigilant physicians will form the first line of any nationwide defense against birth-defect agents, according to Robert W. Miller, M.D., former president of the Teratology Society and chief of the epidemiology branch of the National Cancer Institute.

"Malformations induced by X-ray, German measles (rubella), thalidomide, and inorganic mercury," he has reminded fellow scientists, "were each recognized by an alert practitioner who observed a cluster of cases and then traced the disease to its source."

He recalled instances of fetal defects in the past that were not widely reported at the time. If they had been, as in a nationwide or even worldwide surveillance system, future birth defects could have been prevented.

At Minimata Bay, Japan, for example, a poisoning epidemic was caused by eating fish that had absorbed methylmercury discharged by a factory making vinyl plastic. The outbreak of "Minimata disease" caused cats to go mad and sickened 121 persons, 41 of whom died. Not until several years later was it realized that a parallel epidemic of cerebral palsy had occurred among infants born near Minimata Bay. The frequency had soared from one to twelve palsied children per two hundred births.

"In retrospect," noted Dr. Miller, "it is now clear that Japan was at least ten years ahead of the rest of the world in encountering this pollution problem . . . but neither the congenital nor the adult form of the disease seemed to apply to pollution in other countries, and the reports went largely unnoticed."

Then, fairly recently, methylmercury poisoning struck again—in the United States. The Huckleby family of Alamogordo, New Mexico, bought some seed grain coated with methylmercury-containing fungicide, fed the grain to its hogs (which became ill), butchered the hogs, ate the pork, and came down with Minimata disease. Three of the children suffered extreme brain damage. The mother, seemingly unaffected, was pregnant at the time and later gave birth to a child who appeared to be blind and mentally retarded.

Veterinarians and farmers, as well as M.D.s, might contribute importantly to a birth-defects early warning system. Frequently farm animals and pets are exposed to sizable amounts of chemical agents in air, water, and food that also may be inhaled or consumed by pregnant women.

Thus, a rash of birth defects in baby pigs in Kentucky was believed due to pesticides or growth stimulants used in tobacco cultivation. Lead, from auto exhausts, has been found in grass growing along highways in sufficient concentrations to cause cows eating the vegetation to abort.

Physicians and veterinarians in Missouri have been cooperating in a computerized study of birth defects in human beings, domestic animals, and wild animals. The head of the study, Dr. Carl J. Marienfeld, professor of community health and medical practice at the University of Missouri, has already found that some counties have higher rates of birth defects than others.

In strictly human studies of birth defects there is, according to Dr. Henry A. Schroeder, Dartmouth professor, "a good correlation of certain qualities of municipal water supplies and deaths from congenital abnormalities in the U.S."

In Grand Junction, Colorado, where 150,000 to 200,-000 tons of uranium mine tailings have been used for fill, in concrete slabs and home construction, doctors have noted a rise in birth deformities apparently caused by radioactivity. (In some homes built on the uranium fill, radioactivity readings are above levels permitted in uranium mines. So far, the tailings have been found in 4984 locations in and around Grand Junction; the Colorado Department of Health has recommended removal of the radioactive sand wherever it has been used in or beneath buildings.) Dr. C. Henry Kempe, chairman of the pediatrics department of the School of Medicine, University of Colorado, and Grand Junction pediatrician Robert M. Ross, Jr., also reported to a Congressional subcommittee that birth rates were significantly lower in the area than in the rest of the state. The problem of uranium contamination may exist in nine other Western states where uranium has been mined.

Dr. Robert Miller of the National Cancer Institute has urged that physicians recording stillbirths, miscarriages, and birth defects ask about and note the mother's occupation and any unusual environmental exposure just before or during pregnancy. An example of what might be found:

In pregnancies surveyed recently by Stanford University investigators, women who worked in hospital operating rooms were found to have a miscarriage rate more than three times that of general-duty nurses and physicians. The vapors of anesthetic gases were blamed. Miscarriages occurred in ten of thirty-six pregnancies of operating nurses, but in only three of thirty-four pregnancies of unexposed general-duty nurses. Fourteen of thirty-seven pregnant anesthetists miscarried, but only six of fifty-eight general physicians.

Increased risk of spontaneous abortion, involuntary fertility, and the birth of abnormal children appeared in a concurring survey, disclosed in 1972, covering 80 percent of all women anesthetists in Great Britain. A Danish study at the same time revealed not only more miscarriages among women who worked in operating rooms, but also among the wives of male anesthetists —and an unusually high percentage of females among their babies.

Until the shadowy world of teratogens is fully mapped, caution is the only wise course for the mother-to-be.

"All drugs are suspect," says the March of Dimes' Dr. Virginia Apgar. "Everything from aspirin to zinc oxide to baking soda taken for heartburn."

Many capsules and substances taken routinely fall under the ban: laxatives, pep pills, tranquilizers, any pain reliever, mineral oil, reducing pills, nerve tonic, sleeping pills, vitamin supplements, antibiotics, nose drops, inhalers, suppositories, salves, and ointments.

Nose drops, used to contract the blood vessels of the nose, could also be strong enough to contract blood vessels in the placenta and reduce oxygen and nutrition carried to the fetus.

Too much vitamin K can cause jaundice that may damage the nervous system of the fetus. A great excess of vitamin D taken by the mother may cause mental retardation in the fetus and defects of the heart and bones. This happened in England soon after World War II, when vitamin D supplementation became a fad.

Dr. Apgar, writing in *Word*, suggests that "The array of potential destruction to an unborn child in the average family's medicine chest is far more treacherous" than the menace of the more notorious drugs, such as LSD. She cites a study of 86 California families that revealed a total of 2623 medications in their medicine chests—an average of 30 per family. Only 445, or about one-sixth of these were prescription items—and 99 were entirely without labels.

Of course, "hard" drugs are not hazard-free. Newborn babies of heroin addicts, for example, suffer from withdrawal symptoms during the twenty-four-hour period after birth. If untreated, up to 90 percent may die (death can also occur in the womb if the mother is suddenly withdrawn from heroin). But if they are properly treated, says Richard H. Schwarz, M.D., of the hospital of the University of Pennsylvania, mortality from this cause in otherwise healthy infants should be nil. Treatment usually consists of gradually decreasing dosages of morphine or phenobarbital for the newborn, "the most readily cured of all addicts."

Since the 1964–1965 rubella epidemic and its resulting damage to the unborn, medicine has been pressing its attack on maternal *infections* that directly injure the fetus. Some, like rubella, cause abnormalities in the unborn and therefore are considered teratogens. Others stunt or sicken the fetus without causing deformities, or infect the newborn during birth, as he passes through an infected vagina.

Unlike chemical teratogens, which usually damage the fetus only in early gestation, many infections are a danger for most of the pregnancy.

Among the most obviously preventable of the infections are the venereal diseases. "Yet," says The National Foundation—March of Dimes, "the number of babies born with venereal infections rises with appalling rapidity." (The foundation estimates that "if current trends continue," 1.2 million of today's 4 million fifteen-year-olds will contract VD before they are twenty-five.)

Congenital syphilis in the newborn may cause blistery sores, crippling bone deformities, anemia, liver and spleen enlargement—or it may be hidden, only to result in blindness and other disastrous damage in later years. However, it can be prevented by treating and curing the mother, with antibiotics, before the eighteenth week of pregnancy; after that time, the disease can cross the placenta and affect the baby.

Gonorrhea infects the newborn as he passes through the birth canal during delivery. Gonorrheal

conjunctivitis, which rapidly produces ulcers and per-
foration of the cornea of the baby's eyes, can result in
scarring and blindness. Tetracycline ointment, used
to prevent the infection, has not always proved effective. But the disease can be prevented if the mother is
tested for gonorrhea shortly before delivery, and
cured with antibiotics.

Strep infections of the vagina can produce no symptoms in the mother and still be disastrous for the baby
who becomes infected during birth. A group of investigators at Children's Hospital, Denver, found Group
B streptococcal infections in almost 5 percent of
women giving birth. In 1971, they said, streptococcal
infections accounted for at least 8 percent of all newborn deaths in Colorado.

Working with two Denver obstetrical groups, the
Children's Hospital team has developed a preventive
approach. Vaginal cultures are taken at the expectant
mother's first visit to the doctor, at three months' gestation, six months, shortly before delivery, and at
delivery. "When we find group B [streptococci] prenatally—four in forty so far—we treat the mother with
oral or intramuscular penicillin, or oral erythromy-
cin," reported Dr. Ralph A. Franciosi. "And we culture the husband, and if he's positive we treat both.
We're finding that we can treat and clear the maternal
vagina with no risk to the mother, and therefore the
baby will no longer be at risk from this problem."

More tests to detect teratogenic infections seem to
be in the offing for expectant mothers.

At the University of Alabama Medical Center, all
pregnant women are now tested for at least four infections known to endanger the unborn baby: rubella
virus, toxoplasmosis, syphilis, and cytomegalovirus
(CMV).

Dr. John L. Sever of the National Institute of

Neurological Diseases and Stroke has suggested that physicians and testing laboratories give special attention to three teratogenic virus diseases—rubella, CMV, and herpes simplex—because these can possibly be prevented by vaccines or treated.

Among all birth-defect-causing diseases, perhaps none has gained public attention as quickly as toxoplasmosis. Until recently, the parasitic disease was known only to physicians and researchers. But in 1971 came news of a scientific finding about it that shocked mothers and mothers-to-be: blame for a baby's birth defect in some cases could be placed on the head of the family cat, which can be a carrier of toxoplasmosis and transmit it to humans.

A common infection that for most adults seems no worse than a cold and is often assumed to be one, toxoplasmosis at one time or another has struck at least 25 percent of U.S. adults (who carry antibodies and are thus presumed to be immune from further attacks). But if it is contracted by a pregnant woman, it can cause extensive brain damage to the fetus, malformation of the head, fatal illness, or blindness. According to The National Foundation—March of Dimes, one in every four thousand newborn babies shows defects due to prenatal infection by toxoplasmosis; about one in one thousand appears to be normal, but is infected and may develop serious neurological problems later in life.

In the absence of a vaccine or treatment for the disease, precautionary measures have been recommended for any prospective or expectant mother who has a cat. These include a blood test to see if the woman is already immune; an analysis of the cat's feces by a veterinarian to determine if the cat is infected, and rubber-gloved emptying of the cat's litter box daily.

Informed cat lovers have been quick to point to scientific opinion that rare or raw meat is still the chief route of infection for humans as well as cats. (Heating all meat to at least 140 degrees throughout kills the toxoplasmosis organism.) But what toxoplasmosis-aware expectant mother, out for an evening at a friend's house, would now cuddle her hosts' friendly feline? Avoiding a cat is easy. The test of prudent pregnancy will come at dinnertime, when she faces a tempting plate of rare sirloin and whipped (blight-free??) potatoes.

CHAPTER

IV

Nourishing the Unborn

The revolution in obstetrics is largely a story of steady progress.

Not so the most revolutionary and perhaps most important chapter of that story. For this is a tale of gross error, of neglect and conflict, persisting over decades and not yet fully rectified.

In short, many if not most U.S. doctors have been mismanaging the nutrition of pregnant women. This is the finding of the prime U.S. authority on this subject, the Committee on Maternal Nutrition of the Food and Nutrition Board, National Research Council, National Academy of Sciences. Its landmark report (1970), wrote chairman Robert E. Shank, M.D., in *Nutrition Today*, "clearly shows the need for a significant change in the way physicians and others now view the pregnant woman's diet. It focuses on the need for a new approach . . . and suggests abandoning many current practices widely accepted as safe."

If followed, the recommendations of the report conceivably could save thousands of American babies each year from low birthweight, prematurity, and resultant mental retardation, severe illness, or death.

Among the standard practices condemned in the panel's report, *Maternal Nutrition and the Course of Pregnancy*, are:

•Rigid restriction of weight gain in pregnancy. (For a time the accepted range of weight gain was ten to fourteen pounds. A popular 1972 medical textbook recommended a seventeen-pound gain.) Twenty-four pounds is more like it, says the committee.

•Low-salt diets as a routine measure.

•Routine use of diuretics. (In 1972, 60 to 70 percent of all U.S. pregnant women received diuretics, estimates Frederick P. Zuspan, M.D., chief of obstetrics, Pritzker School of Medicine, University of Chicago.)

"There has been a return to older concepts regarding nutrition in pregnancy," explains Dr. Philip L. White, director of the department of foods and nutrition of the American Medical Association. Some of the condemned practices have been applied for fifty years; weight restriction began in the 1920s. Widespread use of diuretics in pregnancy became popular in the 1950s. "In the past, the physician has been extremely conservative about caloric intake. He has too frequently used sodium restriction and diuretics to prevent some of the edema [swelling] that seems to occur. So the recent efforts have been to try to get the obstetrician to approach nutrition in pregnancy in a manner which will provide optimum nutrition and avoid emphasis on weight control."

What's so bad about weight restriction in pregnancy?

At Dr. White's suggestion, I sought answers from Robert M. Kark, chief of the renal and nutrition sections of Rush Presbyterian–St. Luke's Medical Center in Chicago. He is also a member of the Food and Nutrition Board of the National Research Council.

"I don't think weight gain in pregnancy should be limited to any set figure or range," Dr. Kark told me. "I don't mind the twenty-four pound suggestion of the 1970 Research Council report. But I wouldn't place any restrictions on it. Most women tend to put on the proper weight for them. Now, if someone's going to gain one hundred pounds, that's crazy, you know. But if you have a great big woman who's six foot three, she's not going to be gaining the same kind of weight as the girl who's five feet and slight. It's an individual matter. All I'm saying is that restricting weight should not be part of the general practice of obstetrics. And too many obstetricians are still trying to reduce women's weight during pregnancy. That's nonsense. It's clearly been shown that women on reducing diets in pregnancy have much higher illness rates with their babies."

Diet restriction was thought to prevent large babies and thus make for easier deliveries; weight control and low-salt diets were believed preventive against toxemia of pregnancy, one of the chief dangers to mother and baby. But neither of these theories proved true.

Toxemia of pregnancy, explains Dr. Kark, is a blanket term for a condition in which there is high blood pressure, protein in the urine, and abnormal retention of fluid. The great fear regarding toxemia—which affects 7 percent of first pregnancies in the United States—is that it will turn into eclampsia—convulsions and coma followed by death for 5 percent of the women who experience it, death for 30 percent of their unborn babies.

But there are three different kinds of toxemia of pregnancy, explains Dr. Kark. One kind is a condition, occurring only in pregnancy and with no apparent underlying cause, known as preeclampsia. Another is renal (kidney) disease in pregnancy: "If you enter pregnancy with renal disease and at the end of pregnancy you're sick, you'll be diagnosed as having toxemia." Another is high blood pressure in pregnancy, which may just be a continuation of a prepregnancy condition.

"Why shouldn't low-salt diets be used in pregnancy?" I asked Dr. Kark.

"The situation is very simple," he said. "As the mother and child grow, the tissues grow with them and there's an *increased* requirement for sodium. So the whole idea of starting off at the beginning of pregnancy with a low-salt diet can do nothing but harm, and tends to *produce* toxemia of pregnancy. Where studies have been made of pregnant women on a low-salt diet and those not so restricted, the instance of toxemia was higher among the low-salt group. These findings were published in *Lancet* [Britain's leading medical journal] fifteen years ago."

Later in pregnancy, if toxemia develops, Dr. Kark does advise a low-salt diet. "Once a patient has edema, she has to go on a low-salt diet, because she obviously has a disturbance and needs to reduce the sodium that causes fluid retention. But you precipitate disease by putting women on low-salt diets when they don't need it, especially when the baby's growing. That's very bad."

Dr. Kark does not even recommend use of low-salt diets throughout pregnancy for women with high blood pressure.

In such cases, says Dr. Kark, "doctors tend to take the sodium down right away. That does nothing but harm.

"We make sure such a patient gets enough antihypertension drugs while we keep the sodium in the diet up. You have to have some sodium for the uterus that's growing, for the placenta that's growing, and for the *baby*. What are you going to do with him? Kill him?"

What's the matter with diuretics in pregnancy?

"The routine use of diuretics without specific clinical indications is unwise," says the National Research Council report, *Maternal Nutrition and the Course of Pregnancy*. Furthermore, "The widespread practice of routinely restricting salt intake and at the same time prescribing diuretics is of doubtful value in preventing preeclampsia and is potentially dangerous."

"Diuretics prevent edema but nothing else," points out the University of Chicago's Dr. Frederick P. Zuspan, one of the nation's leading experts on toxemia of pregnancy, "and they may disturb the homeostatic mechanisms during pregnancy."

He uses diuretics only to control chronic high blood pressure and treats mild preeclampsia with bed rest (the patient lying on her side, which promotes the rapid loss of excess fluid) and a high-protein, salt-restricted diet.

Even if eclampsia occurs, Zuspan refrains from using diuretics, which are commonly used in conventional treatment along with depressants, barbiturates, antihypertensives, tranquilizers, narcotics, and other medications.

Instead, he tells his medical students with a smile, "since 1962 we have given only magnesium sulfate to the patient, barbiturates to the nursing staff, tranquilizers to the faculty, and narcotics to the students. Hence, everybody has some medication and the patient is then better off."

Science and authorities aside, the figure-conscious American woman may not want to accept the liberal weight gain recommended by the National Research Council. For, if she does eat well and gains twenty-four pounds, she will be left with four to eight pounds of solid weight gain after the birth of her baby and the loss of tissues and fluids.

Mother Nature has a special purpose for adding these extra pounds, suggests Dr. Charles U. Lowe of the National Institute of Child Health and Human Development, who points out that it may be a natural way of providing a reserve for breast-feeding—which requires one thousand calories per day. Even an excess gain of twenty-four pounds, remaining after birth, could be used up in just three and one-half months of normal breast-feeding.

Far more important than cosmetic considerations is the effect on the unborn baby of an ample maternal diet. Far too many American babies are undernourished before birth, and consequently are born prematurely or small for their gestational age.

"The proportion of low-birthweight infants," said *Maternal Nutrition and the Course of Pregnancy*, "remains high . . . and appears to be rising."

These babies are at high risk. Prematurity, a frequent result of fetal starvation, contributes directly or indirectly to more than 50 percent of deaths during the first month of life, according to Denis Cavanaugh, M.D., chairman of obstetrics, St. Louis University School of Medicine. The premature baby is thirty times as likely to die as the full-term infant, he adds, and survivors are more prone to mental retardation, neurologic diseases, and blindness.

"We can infer from the published data of Dr. Tom Brewer," says Dr. Lowe, "that a nutritious diet producing a generous weight gain during pregnancy can, in fact, remarkably reduce the incidence of low birthweight. In fifteen hundred pregnancies among a low-income group of women, the prematurity rate [birth-weight below six pounds is generally accepted as a rule-of-thumb indication of prematurity] was 2.2 percent; and even among 318 primipara (first-birth women) from fourteen to twenty-one years of age, the rate was only 2.8 percent. These numbers should be compared with the national average of 8.2 percent [1968] and 15 percent in low-income black women.

"These conclusions challenge the conventional wisdom, which demands constraint on weight gain by caloric restriction, a limitation of salt intake, and use of saline diuretics. None of these were used in the Brewer series.

"If these observations are confirmed in other and larger series, we will be in a position to explain what to date has confounded those epidemiologists studying infant mortality rates and prematurity rates. Why have we failed to reduce infant mortality as effectively as other modern nations and why is our prematurity rate rising, a factor of life in no other advanced nation?

"The answer may well lie in our prenatal regimens. It looks as if we can make real progress on both questions merely by feeding pregnant women."

Dr. Denis Cavanaugh, writing on "The Challenge of Prematurity" in *Medical World News,* concurs: "There is much to suggest that, if the poor were provided with a well-balanced diet including high-quality proteins, fruits, and vegetables, the prematurity rate would be reduced."

Cavanaugh points to the same evidence cited by Lowe: "In this respect it is interesting that Dr. Tom Brewer, running a county prenatal clinic serving indigent women in Richmond, California [but also serving an equal number of nonpoor—Ed.] has reduced the incidence of low birthweight infants (premature and pseudopremature, or undersized full-term babies). . . . His daily dietary instructions include a quart of milk, two eggs, one or two servings of meat or fish, one or two helpings of green vegetables, two or three slices of whole wheat bread, one glass of fruit juice, and one pat of vitamin-A-enriched margarine. This is surely a diet anyone can afford." (Low-cost, high-protein foods such as beans are specified by the clinic for those who cannot afford meat.)

Who is this Dr. Brewer, whose results, confirmed by a recently completed HEW study, can only be described as astounding?

He is a Ralph Nader of obstetrics, a crusader "dashing about in all directions," as one detractor put it, "on a pregnant white horse." For nearly a decade Brewer has been noisily scolding his fellow obstetricians for their adherence to prenatal regimens he was convinced were dangerous: routine low-salt diets, diuretics, and low weight gain. He blames such practices for much of U.S. malnutrition during pregnancy among rich and poor, which he claims is annually responsible for the deaths of more than 30,000 infants and birth defects suffered by more than 200,000 children. Maternal malnutrition, he believes, is responsible for most mental retardation in this country.

He is the founder of two organizations of consumers which promote his views: NAG (Nutrition Action Group), which disseminates nutritional concepts at prenatal clinics and before interested groups in San Francisco, and SPUN (Society for the Protection of the Unborn Through Nutrition), a new, similar organization based in Chicago.

Now in his mid-forties, of medium build, with close-cropped brown hair and conservative dress, Dr.

Brewer does not have the appearance of a revolutionary. Says a friend, Dr. Robert Mendelsohn, former medical director of Head Start: "He's the straightest-looking guy you can imagine, business suit, mild manner. But in the softest, most placid voice you can imagine, he says the most outrageous and bloodcurdling things about his fellow physicians."

Among the targets at which Brewer directs a continuous stream of angry comments and correspondence is the American Medical Association. Yet the AMA's circumspect nutritional expert, Dr. Philip White, told me: "I can't disagree with what Dr. Brewer says, although I feel he is prone to exaggerate to make his point. His hangup is the obstetrician who for the most part pays only lip service to the concept of good nutrition before and during pregnancy. . . . I think the medical profession has not done a very commendable job in recognizing the role of nutrition in pregnancy. And Dr. Brewer obviously is very much concerned about this."

"Dr. Brewer sounds like a wild man," I had remarked to the National Research Council's Dr. Robert Kark, one of the nation's foremost experts on maternal nutrition. "He is," admitted Dr. Kark. "He's a fanatic. All the obstetricians have gone one way, which was incorrect. And now he's overreacting to it. That's my opinion. But I think he's in the right direction."

"My point of view is not popular with most U.S. and most West European obstetrical authorities and practitioners," admits Dr. Brewer. "I see a direct and causal relationship between malnutrition during pregnancy and the development of five common clinical disorders: metabolic toxemia of late pregnancy, abruptio placentae [premature detachment of the placenta, a major cause of fetal damage and maternal hemorrhage], severe maternal-fetal and newborn infections, severe maternal anemias, and a high percentage of low birthweight infants. I think the evidence is strong that a high percentage of first trimester spontaneous abortions and congenital anomalies (birth defects), including central-nervous-system-damaged infants, are also causally related to maternal-fetal malnutrition."

In a recent letter to a friend ("one of the very few obstetrics-gynecology people in academic medicine who will even communicate with me"), he related how his present views and practices evolved:

Had I always listened to the advice of my elders, I would never have done a bit of creative thinking or research in this field. As a medical student at Tulane University in 1950 I was taught (as medical students are still being taught today, 1972): "The cause of toxemia of pregnancy is unknown . . . and among the most likely theories is that of a primary utero-placental ischemia" [blood deficiency caused by constriction or obstruction of blood vessels].

I was taught that there is no evidence that malnutrition during pregnancy can cause diseases of human pregnancy . . . and yet all around me during my last two years at Charity Hospital, New Orleans, my year of internship at Jefferson Davis in Houston and my year of GP residency in rural Louisiana, I was meeting and talking with some of the poorest and most malnourished women and girls in the nation. These poor women suffered in rural Louisiana an incidence of toxemia of 25 percent; they had (and still have in 1972): acute cases of placental separation; severe, life-taking infections; severe anemias, and so many low birthweight and damaged newborns!

And all around me I saw and heard my colleagues shouting at these pregnant poor: "Don't eat . . . lose weight . . . don't eat salt . . . or you'll have fits and die and your baby will die!" During my internship at Jeff Davis, I heard one of my most memorable clues to these problems from the attendings in obstetrics-gynecology who would come in to help us. On many occasions they said: "We don't see these cases of eclampsia, of severe abruptions, etc. in private practice very often. We have to come back here to J.D. to see them."

Why are these poor women and girls such "high risks" I asked over and over . . . and as the years passed and I did more clinical work, the answer became glaringly apparent. From rural Louisiana I went into private general practice in a small town in Fulton, Missouri where toxemia of pregnancy was practically non-existent! Why? Because I had left the poverty-hunger belt of the Deep South, U.S.A. It was here in Missouri that I became convinced of the validity of the opinions of [researchers] M. B. Strauss and Bertha Burke.

In January, 1958, in Fulton, Missouri, I saw Merck, Sharp & Dohme beginning their "hard sell" campaign for saluretic diuretics for use in "toxemia of pregnancy" and for "edema in pregnancy." In May, 1958, I went back to the Deep South, to Miami, Florida and told the chief of obstetrics at Jackson Memorial Hospital that the diuretic promotion was wrong, was covering up the real problems of maternal-fetal malnutrition. I asked for a research fellowship to study the role of malnutrition in toxemia and low birthweight, abruptio, etc. . . . But in 1958 there was no interest in human pregnancy nutrition among our Ob-Gyn academics and no money to study the role of hunger in human reproductive pathology.

During four years at Jackson Memorial (as a resident in obstetrics) I began to recognize the B.S. which still passes for scientific knowledge and fact in this field; it is piled up many miles high and buried centuries deep. I went to national conventions of ACOG [American College of Obstetricians and Gynecologists] for four years in a row and talked with all of the "old men" of U.S. Ob-Gyn with the least bit of interest in "toxemia of pregnancy" and I learned that not a single one of them knew a damned thing about it!

What was totally unperceived by our Ob-Gyn experts was the glaring fact of hypovolemia [abnormally decreased blood-fluid volume] with the associated hemoconcentration [blood concentration] and hypoalbuminemia [low content in the blood of albumin, a protein constituent of blood serum]. There is reduction of utero-placental blood flow in severe toxemia, but it is secondary to falling blood volume, secondary to a falling serum albumin level, secondary to protein-calorie *dietary deficiency!* I have proved this on the clinical level with pregnant humans in many different ways. . . .

I have come to see that we are confronted with another of the body's homeostatic or self-righting mechanisms: the renin-angio-tension-aldosterone mechanism which functions to protect the integrity of the maternal blood volume. You have perhaps already grasped how wrong it has been all these years to prescribe low-salt diets and salt diuretics to the pregnant woman who has a stress to maintain an expanded blood volume throughout the last half of gestation" [blood volume is elevated considerably in a normal pregnancy—Ed.].

In Merced County, California, in 1970, *a physician* starved a young Mexican-American woman into complications, i.e. hypovolemic shock and a low birthweight at term [delivery] infant—and the infant suffered profound neonatal [newborn] hypoglycemia [lack of blood sugar, the fuel of brain cells] and is now obviously mentally retarded. I will not say her doctor did it with malice or even deliberately—but *he did it!* He told the young woman she could gain only 15 pounds—and she gained from 112 to 125 pounds—and he told her to avoid milk and eggs, to avoid salt . . . and for three months he had her take a diuretic pill, or two, every day. This infant was 16 inches long and weighed four pounds, 15 ounces at term. In my nutrition project in Pittsburg with her second pregnancy she ate well and gained from 112 to 162; her second baby weighed 9 pounds, 12 ounces and was 22 inches long (same father). We will continue to have iatrogenic [doctor-caused] malnutrition in human prenatal care until the ACOG recognizes the role of malnutrition in damaging mother and fetus—until we set up some national nutrition standards for human pregnancy nutrition—until we teach medical students, interns, residents and teaching staffs of obstetrics-gynecology the basic principles of applied, scientific nutrition for practice in human prenatal care. . . .

For many years, partly because he refused to use control groups of patients who would receive standard care, Brewer could not get grants. He still has none. But in 1972–1973, the National Institute of Child Health and Human Development conducted a $107,-000 analysis of his successful experiment in nutrition during pregnancy, a study covering seven thousand hospital admissions, 1965–1970.

"They have already learned," wrote Brewer to his friend, "that pregnant patients in my project gain more weight and have larger babies than in practically any other study in history." [The average birthweight for black babies in the project is 7.4 pounds while the national average for blacks is only 5.9; in two counties in Mississippi where the average black birthweight is about 5 pounds, infant mortality is greater than one child in ten.]

"In this study," continued Brewer, "we have exploded so many myths and false assumptions:

"1. We have exploded the 'genetic theory' about infant birthweight and length (used to explain the fact that non-white babies are usually smaller than whites).

"2. We have exploded the myth that the placenta is a parasite (that the baby gets what it needs no matter what).

"3. We have exploded the myth about the teenager or the young primigravida [first pregnancy]—both considered high risk because of their age, the 'tight uterus' [of the first pregnancy, used to explain its higher risk], the primary 'utero-placental ischemia' [hardening of arteries in the uterus as the basic cause of a poorly nourished placenta], etc.

"4. We have explained why women in low-income groups and in minority groups are 'high-risks' by feeding them and removing them from such a category.

"5. We have shown the harm in drugs, in low-calorie, low-salt diets, in blind weight control—by throwing them out of the prenatal clinic and observing superior reproductive results without them.

"6. We have thus offered a scientific explanation for failure of our nation to reduce the incidence of low birthweight babies, by reducing these rates with scientific nutrition education and practices.

"7. We have been demonstrating the role of maternal-fetal malnutrition in central-nervous-system-damaged infants by preventing them."

Brewer, who believes that a normal, healthy weight gain in pregnancy is usually about thirty to thirty-five pounds, points to evidence gathered by the Collaborative Study of Cerebral Palsy carried on by the National Institute of Neurological Disease and Stroke. The $100-million-plus survey, of more than 55,000 deliveries in fourteen leading U.S. medical centers, showed a direct relationship between maternal weight gain in pregnancy and birthweight, length, and lessened neurological damage to infants. Women who gained thirty-six pounds or more during pregnancy had only about one-third the number of brain-damaged children and one-third the number of low birthweight infants as those who gained zero to fifteen pounds.

Most of the plump ladies in the survey ate enough of the nutrients essential for a good pregnancy, Brewer concludes, and many of the zero-to-fifteen-pound gainers did not. He adds that a mother-to-be of course can gorge herself, gain too much weight, and develop toxemia or produce a low birthweight baby "if she lacks adequate proteins of high biological quality."

Plenty of protein is needed during pregnancy, not only for growth of bone and muscle in the fetus, but also for adequate production of brain cells in the baby. There is mounting evidence, according to foremost authority Dr. Myron Winick of Columbia University, that a baby seriously deprived of protein before birth and in the first six months of life will develop fewer brain cells; his brain will be stunted for life. This may help to explain why mental retardation is so common among the malnourished poor. The President's Committee on Mental Retardation estimates the mental retardation rate among the poor to be two or three times the national average, which is about 3 percent. Pediatrician E. Perry Crump of Meharry Medical College found 14 percent of indigent children treated at the college's teaching hospital to be mentally retarded, and estimates that the rate may reach 33 percent in certain areas of extreme poverty. (Mental retardation caused by malnutrition after infancy, however, may be reversible by protein feeding.)

Anemia is a common threat today to U.S. pregnancies, according to the AMA's Dr. Philip White, because a good many American women enter pregnancy with a deficiency of iron. Yet it is easily correctible with prescribed iron pills. Without sufficient iron, the blood lacks enough red blood cells to carry plenteous oxygen from the mother's lungs to the cells of her baby. Deprived of oxygen, the baby grows more slowly and not as well. When he is born, even after a full nine months' gestation, he is smaller than average.

Exactly the same phenomenon occurs when the mother smokes cigarettes, declares Dr. Maria Delivoria-Papadopoulas, a University of Pennsylvania clinical researcher studying maternal-fetal blood flow. "We are finding," she told me, "that babies of smoking mothers are being born small, that there are more miscarriages, stillbirths, and newborn deaths and breathing difficulties. Instead of oxygen, the babies in utero are breathing carbon monoxide!"

Dr. Delivoria-Papadopoulas, a youthful, widely respected investigator, stresses that oxygen is even more important than food in the nutrition of the baby. Deprived of oxygen for only a few minutes, the cells of the body begin to die. No food can be utilized by the body without oxygen.

Dr. Delivoria-Papadopoulas and associates found (by sampling umbilical-cord blood of babies at birth) that babies of smoking mothers have nearly four times the carbon monoxide in their blood as babies of nonsmokers. In babies whose mothers smoked two packs of cigarettes a day until four to six hours before delivery, 9.4 percent of the oxygen-carrying capacity of the blood was blocked by carbon monoxide, as compared with 0.7 to 2.5 percent in the babies of nonsmoking women.

From her studies, this investigator has concluded that the number of cigarettes that can be safely smoked by a pregnant woman is *zero*. High-traffic areas of cities, such as downtown, and also industrial sections, produce air pollution that results in much the same effect as smoking. They are high-risk areas for pregnant women, as are rooms and automobiles in which others are smoking.

Curiously, rest periods and appropriate exercise such as long walks are important to the *nutrition* of the fetus. For they help to ensure good blood flow from mother to placenta to baby, and a generous supply of oxygen fuel to all the fetal cells.

Until recently, U.S. nutritionists believed that the average American woman entering pregnancy needed no supplemental vitamins. Of all things, the Pill has changed that. "Recent studies," says the AMA's Dr. White, "have shown that birth-control pills cause an increased requirement for certain vitamins. This may cause some women to enter pregnancy with a shortage of these vitamins, one in particular being folic acid, one of the B-complex vitamins.

"One effect of a folic acid deficiency," adds Dr. White, "is megaloblastic anemia, in which the blood cells become larger than normal but never completely mature, and therefore don't function efficiently. Whether this is related to the common disorder, anemia of pregnancy, needs researching, as does the relationship of the Pill to increased vitamin requirements. (Vitamin B_6[pyridoxine] is another vitamin thought to be affected.)"

Tufts University pediatrics chairman Dr. Sydney S. Gellis has warned of the dangers of too many vitamin pills during pregnancy. "Unfortunately," he remarked, "vitamins are looked on as foodstuffs, so pregnant women tend to overdose with them."

CHAPTER

V

Surgery Before Birth

The date is circa 1980.

The scene: the operating room of a university hospital. On the table, draped with green cloths for surgery, is a young woman in midpregnancy, her abdomen still only gently rounded. Inside her womb is a baby who would be doomed save for the operation that will occur today.

Through methods of detection refined in the late 1970s, it has been learned that the unborn baby has a diaphragmatic hernia—a hole in the diaphragm, the wall of muscle that supports the lungs. The hole is so big that the baby's small intestines have pushed through from below and filled much of the interior of the chest. Unless this flaw is corrected, the tiny human, now thriving, will be born with undeveloped lungs and will die within the first ten minutes of its life outside the womb.

The surgeon cuts through the mother's abdominal wall, then the wall of the uterus, until he at last reaches the paper-thin, fluid-filled amniotic sac that holds the baby.

Gently the surgeon manipulates the sleeping baby in its watery cradle, until its abdomen is snug against the operative opening. Then, in an oval pattern, he sews the baby's belly to the wall of its mother's abdomen at the point of incision. Within the stitched oval, operating with the aid of magnifying glasses and the tiniest of instruments, he deftly cuts through the amniotic sac, makes an opening in the baby's abdomen, tenderly pulls the escaping intestine back into the abdominal cavity, and sews shut the gaping hole in the diaphragm muscle.

Now retreating, the surgeon closes the tissue doors he has just opened, releasing the baby from its stitches, repairing the delicate amniotic sac while not neglecting to collect and replace any amniotic fluid that has been spilled.

In less than an hour the operation is over. A young life has been saved by means of an operation undreamed of a few years ago.

This procedure and other major surgery on the human fetus is predicted by Dr. Karlis Adamsons, M.D., Ph.D., of New York's Mount Sinai School of Medicine, a pioneering investigator and authority in the field. It was Dr. Adamsons, together with Dr. Vincent J. Freda, who in 1963 first opened the amniotic sac to perform an operation on a human fetus.

The fetus, 27½ weeks old, was dying of anemia from Rh disease. A new technique of treating the condition had just been developed by Dr. A. W. Liley of New Zealand, in which concentrated red blood cells were injected by catheter through the mother's abdomen, the uterine wall, the amniotic tissue, and finally into the abdominal cavity of the fetus, which would thereafter gradually absorb them. The new method, subsequently refined and now the standard treatment, had at first only indifferent success when emulated in other countries. And so Freda and Adamsons, both then at Columbia-Presbyterian Hospital in New York, opted for a more direct method of getting fresh blood into the dying baby.

They made an incision in the mother's abdomen, located one foot of the fetus, cut into the uterus and amniotic sac, pulled out the foot, and kept it outside the mother's body for two and one-half hours so that they could perform an exchange transfusion through the artery of the leg to give the baby a complete refill of rich new blood.

Although this operation and four others which followed were unsuccessful in correcting the aftereffect of the long-standing fetal anemia, some of the pregnancies continued for as long as eight weeks after the initial surgery. And they paved the way for future successes in fetal surgery.

In 1965, at the University of Puerto Rico School of Medicine, Dr. Stanley H. Asensio used a modified Freda-Adamsons approach to transfuse blood directly into the exposed upper leg of a fetus. The result was a much-improved baby born three weeks later by Cesarean section; today that child is a normal, healthy schoolgirl. Since then Dr. Asensio has successfully performed a similar procedure on a twenty-week-old fetus weighing just over a pound, and has removed another completely from the womb for half an hour before returning it for an eventual normal birth. At other major medical centers around the world, investigators operating on fetal lambs, monkeys, and other animals are preparing the way for more intricate surgery on the unborn human.

"Obviously," Dr. Adamsons told me in a recent interview, "there are very few conditions that have to be treated surgically prior to the birth of the child. And some are so difficult to diagnose that one would not even try. So the field will not become of *major* interest to the clinician."

Yet Dr. Adamsons foresees several possible needed applications of fetal surgery, in addition to the correction of fetal anemia and Rh disease.

"Congenital heart disease would be an ideal condition to treat in the fetal stage," he says. "You don't have to worry about the lung, about stopping respiration, because a fetus does not use its lungs anyway. No heart-lung machine, impracticable in newborns anyhow, is needed; the mother's body serves that purpose. The operation does not have to be hurried. And also, early in gestation the fetus is much more tolerant than the newborn is to transient interruption in circulation.

"The cardiovascular surgeon would have to be reeducated a great deal to think of correcting defects like ventricular septal defect [a hole between the left and right sides of the heart] or transposition of great vessels, which could probably be done best in the fetal stage, though you do have to consider the risks of premature delivery, infection of the amniotic cavity, ultraprolonged exposure of the fetus to environment and contamination."

At the present time, diagnosis is the greatest obstacle to fetal surgery. But some congenital heart abnormalities, including the blue-baby condition, can now be diagnosed before birth. A sensor attached to an electrocardiograph is placed on the mother's abdomen and picks up signals from the baby's heart. Certain conditions reveal themselves by characteristic tracings on the electrocardiogram.

Dr. William Berenberg, former president of the

American Academy for Cerebral Palsy, has suggested that "perhaps the optimal time for the correction of spina bifida performed outside the uterus will soon be somewhere in the second trimester, after which the fetus will be returned to the uterus."

Surgery might serve as a monitoring function, Dr. Adamsons has proposed, in cases where a grave birth defect is suspected. Early in pregnancy the uterus could be opened and the fetus inspected, then replaced if normal. This would be an alternative to blind therapeutic abortions, which frequently sacrifice one or more perfectly normal fetuses for every abnormal fetus aborted.

A variant of this would be the placing of devices in the fetus to measure biologic functions such as temperature, blood alkalinity, and heartbeat, and to transmit the information to monitoring equipment. Already, in animal experiments, such "bugs" are relaying information on the condition of the unborn.

At many research centers, experimental surgery on unborn animals (which dates back to 1918) is done only to learn more about the development of the fetus and its abnormalities, and thus prepare the way for better prenatal diagnosis, treatment, and prevention of birth defects. There is little or no thought of developing these techniques for surgery on the unborn human. However, since 1966 Dr. J. Alex Haller, Jr., has headed a research and training program at Johns Hopkins Children's Center geared toward eventual human fetal surgery. "We look upon this," Dr. Haller has said, "as the new frontier in surgery."

Haller explains that the surgeons at the center first operate on unborn animals to create the kinds of abnormalities that sometimes occur in human fetuses— defects in the heart, lungs, diaphragm, intestines, and other parts.

Then the investigators seek ways to *diagnose* the condition in utero—sometimes by analyzing electrocardiograms of the fetus, or oxygen and body chemicals in the amniotic fluid, or X rays and ultrasound pictures.

A fairly common birth defect, for example, is intestinal atresia, in which a secion of the intestine is entirely missing. Research surgeons at Johns Hopkins create the condition in an unborn lamb simply by operating and tying off a portion of the intestine. Then they seek to diagnose it. They inject dye into the amniotic fluid surrounding the unborn lamb. Since the fetus normally drinks and excretes this fluid, the dye shows up on an X-ray picture concentrated inside the lamb at the site of the blockage.

Then the surgeons reopen the uterus and the lamb, eliminate the blocked area, and join the intestine in order to restore normal function.

If the lamb heals without complications and goes on to birth at its regular due date, the surgery is considered a success. (The effect on its mother is minimal.)

Dr. Haller explains that this condition can be operated upon at birth in the newborn baby, but it's risky. Since the baby receives no oral nourishment because of his blocked gut, he may not be able to withstand the operation. Often, too, there is a delay in diagnosing the blockage after birth. If surgery can be done before birth, the baby suffers no interruption of nourishment; he is fed from his mother's blood, recovers rapidly, and is born healed and happy.

Somewhat similar but more critical is the problem of a baby born with a severe heart deformity. Open-heart operations with the use of heart-lung machines aren't feasible in the newborn because the baby's heart is too small; the equipment gets in the way of the operation. An alternative procedure is to pack the baby in ice during the operation to lower metabolism, thus preventing oxygen starvation of the tissues. But it's an extreme and potentially hazardous procedure.

Some surgery before birth, indicated by improved diagnostic methods, could prevent abnormalities from developing, says Dr. Haller. An example: the tubes draining the kidneys of an unborn baby may be blocked. Until a few weeks before birth, this presents no problem, since the mother's kidneys remove the wastes from the blood. However, ten to fifteen weeks before birth, the baby's kidneys have already started to form urine. If the drainage tubes are blocked, the kidneys may eventually be destroyed. And then the baby's sole hope for survival is a kidney transplant shortly after birth. But an operation on the unborn baby could eliminate the blockage and restore normal function to the tubes and kidneys.

Frequently hydrocephalus, one of the worst birth defects, is also caused by a tube blockage. This, too, should be treated before birth. And it could be done surgically, says Dr. Adamsons, without even opening the uterus.

"I'm looking for such cases myself," says Dr. Adamsons. "This would be an exciting opportunity." Dr. Adamsons would probably team up with an experimental neurosurgeon to do the operation, although, he admits, "I have more experience with fetal brain surgery than any neurosurgeon I know."

Hydrocephalus, explains Dr. Adamsons, is commonly caused when a viral infection of the fetus blocks a tube draining cerebrospinal fluid (manufactured in brain cavities) from the brain into the spinal column. (Some cases are also caused by obstructions in tubes between brain cavities.) As more fluid is produced in the brain, the pressure builds up, displacing and destroying brain tissue itself. The pressure eventually causes the baby's head to expand.

"It would be a very simple operation," says Dr. Adamsons. "Your instrument would be a needle that detaches after insertion, leaving a cannula [tube] with a vent that allows fluid to flow from the brain into the amniotic sac. You could just elevate the fetal head against the abdominal wall, and insert the device through the mother's abdominal wall, into the baby's head. Then whenever pressure inside the head rises, it will flow into the amniotic fluid and the fetus will not develop brain damage.

"After birth, a permanent shunt can be emplaced as is now done to carry fluid from the brain into the abdominal cavity, where it is absorbed, or into a major blood vessel. (Or the obstruction may have cleared and a shunt would not be needed.) You know, at present, most shunts are emplaced when the brain is very destroyed by hydrocephalic development."

How soon will the first of any of these operations take place in humans?

"We feel," says Dr. Adamsons, "that the field of prenatal medicine has extraordinary opportunities. But society's priorities often determine whether a field moves ahead or not, whether it attracts investigators and funds.

"Right now we are more preoccupied with the issues of overpopulation, with quantity control. And once that problem is resolved there will be a great interest in quality control. More attention will be focused on diagnostic and therapeutic possibilities in the prenatal period.

"That does not necessarily mean a great deal of fetal surgery. Abortion on demand is becoming accepted generally. The younger generation is growing up with this feeling that pregnancy is not something that you have to be plagued with if you did not seek it; you can terminate it at will. If this is accepted for social or elective reasons, the same kind of reasoning will probably be applied to a pregnancy where you have some questions about its intactness or normality.

"Let's say a mother has a severe viral infection in early gestation. Instead of being apprehensive for the rest of the pregnancy and then finding out that her newborn baby is deaf or blind, she might decide not to take the risk. If a sample of amniotic fluid revealed evidence of viral infection, her doctor would terminate the pregnancy. Then in two or three months she could begin a new pregnancy."

Would this attitude work against allocation of resources for surgical or medical treatment of the ill fetus?

"It all depends on the guarantees for success. If a specific defect is a condition that's going to be recurring with high frequency in future pregnancies, there may be no particular advantage in getting rid of this pregnancy and starting a new one. But obviously there will be a number of conditions where active interference by the doctor will be needed. For instance, with the mother who has diabetes or prediabetes. Or the mother who has become sensitized to blood group substances. The case in which diagnosis has been missed and it is now too late for an abortion. Or refusal of abortion on moral or religious grounds.

"In these cases the fetus will just have to be treated. There are no two ways about it."

CHAPTER

VI

The Fetus Takes His Medicine

The human fetus is an aquatic creature, swimming gracefully about in a warm amber sea of his own making. The amniotic fluid that bathes him is created by his kidneys, lungs, and sweat glands. At first, when he is very tiny and swimming freely, it serves to cushion him against external blows. As he grows to fill most of the uterine space, it begins to nourish him.

At the age of fourteen weeks or perhaps before, the fetus starts to suck and swallow; he begins to drink the amniotic fluid. The fluid, whose waste has been excreted by the maternal kidneys, contains some protein and sugar and prepares the fetal digestive system for the bigger meals to follow. By the time he is nearly ready to be born, he is drinking up to two pints of fluid per day. And this is nearly the equivalent in food value of four ounces of milk daily.

This known, it is now possible to give medicine orally to an ill fetus. The drug is placed in a syringe like that used for extracting samples of amniotic fluid, and injected through the abdominal wall of the mother and into the amniotic sac. The fetus drinks the drug-tinctured amniotic fluid and gradually is medicated.

There are other routes of fetal medication. For years doctors have been medicating the fetus accidently. Drugs used to treat the mother seeped across the placental "barrier," sometimes with harmful effect. More recently, points out Sumner J. Yaffee, of the School of Medicine, State University of New York at Buffalo, drugs have been administered to the pregnant woman in order to affect her unborn baby directly. For, he says, "essentially every pharmacologic substance can and does pass from the maternal to the fetal bloodstream."

Some drugs pass rapidly from mother to fetus. In two or three minutes after his mother has inhaled anesthesia containing short-acting barbiturates, a fetus is affected in the same degree as his mother. If she is "put to sleep," so is he. Certain drugs, however, transfer too slowly to have any therapeutic effect.

A third route to the fetus is direct injection. Digitalis, to prevent heart failure, has been added to blood given by intrauterine transfusion to a fetus with severe Rh disease. (Heart failure sometimes occurs from the anemia caused by Rh disease; digitalis improves the contractile force of the heart.)

One of the first examples of medication of the fetus was for the purpose of fighting infection, by administering penicillin to a pregnant woman with syphilis. (See Chapter III.) The main target of the penicillin was the baby, points out Dr. Yaffee. "The mother does not have to be treated *immediately;* but the fetus does. Penicillin, if given before the fourth or fifth month of pregnancy, prevents the infection from spreading to the fetus, and causing a very severe disease with deformities. If given later, it arrests the disease in both mother and child but doesn't prevent deformities."

In animal experiments at Harvard Medical School, pathologist Thomas J. Gill III and chemist Heinz W. Kunz have found a way to immunize both a fetus and its mother, by administering the shot only to the mother. Says Gill: "By injecting a long-acting vaccine into a human mother during pregnancy, we may be able to provide protection to babies, such as those with cystic fibrosis or other congenital abnormalities, who are particularly susceptible to infections after the birth. The same techniques might possibly be used to counter teratogenic stimuli such as rubella and thus prevent induced congenital anomalies [birth defects caused by infection]."

Calves and lambs in Michigan are already being immunized successfully before birth against two leading killers of young animals—brucellosis (which also causes miscarriages in cattle and undulant fever in humans) and scours. Researchers at Michigan State University inject the vaccines into the amniotic fluid. Immunity (100 percent in the case of scours) is conferred not only in the womb but during the critical early weeks following birth. "Our results," says Dr. Marvis Richardson of the Department of Microbiology and Public Health, "make us feel confident that fetal immunization will someday be common, both on the farm and in the hospital."

Preventing enzyme-deficiency diseases is another reason for fetal medication. Enzymes, many of which are produced in the liver, are catalysts necessary for various chemical processes in the body. And when they are missing the results are often disastrous. Thus, a baby with Pompe's disease cannot metabolize, or burn, glycogen (the chief carbohydrate storage material). Glycogen builds up in the liver and the baby dies of heart failure when three or four months old. Another metabolic disorder is galactosemia, in which the baby cannot convert milk to sugar. Unless the disorder is diagnosed and his diet adjusted, the baby is likely to become mentally retarded or may starve to death.

Galactosemia is one of more than forty metabolic diseases that are potentially diagnosable in utero by examination of a sample of amniotic fluid (amniocentesis). Work is proceeding on a way to remove galactose from the fetal environment and thus possibly prevent the disease from developing.

Metabolic diseases are already being treated both in utero and soon after birth, explains Dr. Henry Nadler, a pioneer of genetic amniocentesis and chief of staff at Children's Memorial Hospital, Chicago. When interviewed for this book, Dr. Nadler was on the trail of the enzyme deficiency responsible for cystic fibrosis, which affects one of every twenty-five hundred white infants (but almost never babies of other races), more than any other genetic disease.

"If you identify it, how will you treat the disease?" I asked him.

"It might be by any of several current methods of enzyme replacement," he answered. "There are attempts being made to replace missing enzymes by infusing the infant with blood plasma (which contains enzymes; even a small amount of enzyme may be enough); by introducing the pure enzyme into the bloodstream; by giving the infant drugs to help him stabilize the little enzyme he has left; or drugs to stimulate production of the enzyme. There are even attempts to transplant enzyme-producing organs into infants."

Dr. Sumner Yaffee has found a way to prevent jaundice, which affects nearly all newborns, by administering phenobarbital daily to the mother beginning two weeks before birth. Barbiturates, he explains, are among a long list of drugs (including insecticides) that stimulate the human liver to produce more enzymes. Among these is the enzyme that helps eliminate bilirubin, the yellow chemical resulting when used-up red blood cells are processed by the body. Most babies develop a mild, harmless degree of jaundice lasting at most only a few days—until their livers have matured enough to remove the excess bilirubin from their blood. But in certain cases, the liver fails in this function, and jaundice builds up to a dangerous level. If untreated, by long exposure of the skin to bright light, or blood transfusions, the acute condition can result in brain damage.

The prenatal phenobarbital treatment, suggests Dr. Yaffee, would probably be administered only in cases where severe jaundice after birth is expected: in Rh disease, sickle-cell anemia, and in cases where a premature birth is anticipated. (The phenobarbital stimulates a generalized increase in production of enzymes, which may not be an entirely good thing.)

The most widespread and valuable use of fetal medication may be in preventing hyaline membrane disease, also known as respiratory distress syndrome. It is by far the major cause of death in newborns. It affects 5 to 10 percent of all newborn infants and at least one-third of those weighing less than four and one-half pounds. The yearly death toll is more than 25,000 in the United States alone. And it is caused by immaturity of the lungs. A vital fatty fluid, mostly lecithin, which normally coats the interior of the lungs, is missing. The absence of this surfactant prevents easy opening of the lungs' tiny air sacs; every breath of the newborn is an effort. Obstructive stringy fibers (hyaline membrane) develop within the lungs.

Researchers for years have tried to avert hyaline membrane disease by speeding up the maturation of the fetal lungs before birth, so that they will produce the necessary surfactant. Researchers in New Zealand have administered steroids to mothers in premature labor, with resultant significant decrease of hyaline membrane disease and an increased survival of infants born at less than thirty-two weeks' gestation. Dr. Mary Ellen Avery of McGill University and Montreal Children's Hospital has had good results in animals and humans with similar therapy, and in May 1973 recommended it for "desperate" situations in which an infant with immature lungs must be delivered before thirty-two weeks. She uses betamethasone, which is similar to a steroid produced by the fetal adrenal cortex. The steroid stimulates the synthesis of lung surfactant, which is not present in the immature fetus.

Dr. Karlis Adamsons of Mount Sinai School of Medicine, in collaboration with two Argentine physicians, hopes to turn the trick with thyroxin. The idea for this method, explained Dr. Adamsons to me, came from observing pregnancies in which mothers have overactive thyroids. Their babies rarely have hyaline membrane disease because, when delivered, they are advanced in maturity by as much as *two or more months.* The maturation is uniform, including skeletal and neurological as well as lung development. Apparently excess thyroxin produced by the mother's overactive thyroid reaches the fetus through the maternal blood supply, speeding up the metabolism of the fetus. All the body processes, including formation of organs, are quickened; it no longer takes nine months to make a baby.

Because a baby doesn't use his lungs until the moment of birth, explains Dr. Adamsons, lung maturity is reached at a later date than that of the heart and circulation in general.

"The newborn kidney and the brain are even less mature at birth than the lungs, but it doesn't matter. The newborn baby doesn't need or use cortical [higher] activity of the brain. Nor is the kidney of great import to the newborn, whereas the lung and circulation are of critical significance. (The circulation is mature enough for exterior survival at twenty weeks' gestation.)"

Many cases of hyaline membrane disease can be anticipated before birth, explains Dr. Adamsons, but prenatal treatment of the condition is nil. Babies likely to be born before thirty-five or thirty-six weeks' gestation are possible victims. These include, among others, babies whose births are induced early to save their lives, such as those affected with the anemia of Rh disease, babies of diabetic mothers, and babies born of mothers with placenta previa.

In the latter condition, the placenta sits in front of the uterine opening and normal delivery cannot take place. "The usual history of placenta previa," explains Dr. Adamsons, "is that sometimes in the last trimester of pregnancy, when the uterine shape and size are changing, the placenta starts to tear. Then bleeding occurs, which is a warning sign to bring the patient into the doctor's office or the hospital. If bleeding increases or labor starts, the doctor is often forced into delivery of a premature baby susceptible to hyaline membrane disease."

Because most newborn deaths and much mental retardation are a direct or indirect result of prematurity (premature babies, for example, are thirty times as likely to die as those of normal gestation), a successful means of preventing prematurity would be of towering significance.

Dr. Adamsons' Argentine collaborators, Drs. Miguel and Maximo Margulies of Buenos Aires, began treatment of human fetuses with thyroxin in 1973. In women with placenta previa before thirty-five weeks, those with Rh disease or diabetes, the procedure was the same: one of the Drs. Margulies would first inject a fine needle through the abdominal wall and into the womb and amniotic sac to obtain fluid for analysis. (The test reveals the relative amount of lecithin being produced by the lungs of the fetus.) With a similar needle, a small amount of thyroxin was injected into the amniotic fluid. During the following days, the fetus drank and excreted and drank again the medicated amniotic fluid, absorbing the thyroxin. His heart rate and other processes speeded up. Additional injections of thyroxin were made as needed, perhaps twice a week, to maintain the desired amount of thyroxin in the amniotic fluid and keep the fetus running toward an early birth.

"We'll check the mother for signs of thyroid overactivity," explained Dr. Adamsons as the tests began, "and the fetus for growth and heart rate. We want to see how the baby tolerates maternal activity. If the fetal heartbeat is doubled or tripled when the mother moves about, for example, it would mean the baby is not getting enough oxygen. With ultrasound pictures, we'll measure the growth of the fetal head. What we anticipate is that the babies will not grow larger in size but will just be more mature. Babies born of hyperthyroid mothers are usually smaller than normal for their gestational age because their metabolic demands are several times that of a normal baby."

Treatment of the baby before birth may in the future include feeding him. Many babies born today are smaller than normal for their gestational age. A small-for-date infant may be the size of a premature yet be nine months along, as mature physically as any normal baby at birth. He has been undernourished in utero and may never recover from this poor start. Like the runt of a litter of puppies, he may be too small all his life. His brain may never develop to its full potential, for cell division before birth has been retarded from lack of nutrients; he actually has fewer brain cells.

This can not always be remedied by feeding the mother better. Disease or other factors may affect the placenta, the blood supply to the uterus, or the umbilical blood flow. A twin or a triplet in utero may be crowded out of its share of food and oxygen. A baby of a diabetic, although large for its gestational age, is stimulated to outgrow its food supply by its own insulin.

"Once accurate diagnosis of fetal undergrowth in utero is possible," says Ernest W. Page, M.D., obstetrics chairman at the University of California School of Medicine, San Francisco, "we are but a few steps from a research effort aimed at supplementary nourishment of the human fetus in utero."

He explains that once diagnosis of uteroplacental insufficiency is made, nutrients would be infused into the amniotic sac. The fetus would thereupon absorb his nutrient supplement while drinking his usual daily amount of amniotic fluid.

"It is reasonable to speculate," adds Dr. Page, "that in the not-too-distant future we will see special centers developed for feeding undergrown infants in utero. The nutrients used will have to be in proper balance, which may vary according to the gestational age of the fetus being supplemented. The research challenges are exciting to contemplate. The goals are realistic, potentially valuable, and certainly possible."

In fetal feeding, as in fetal medication and fetal surgery, diagnosis is the key that will unlock the great breakthroughs of the future.

"Diagnosis and medication of the fetus go hand in hand," a leading geneticist remarked to me. "First you have to know the fetus is sick."

"The techniques of fetal surgery have been worked out," a pediatric surgeon told me. "That's no problem anymore. But how do you know that a fetus has a hole in its heart, or no kidneys? We're all ready to go once the problems of detection are solved."

"As the field of intrauterine diagnosis expands and becomes more sophisticated," predicts Dr. Robert L. Brent of Jefferson Medical College, "there is every reason to believe that the genetic, biochemical, and physical status of every early embryo will be determinable."

Then, he suggests, systematic abortion or treatment of abnormal embryos during the first three months of pregnancy should be adopted as a standard approach to the problem of congenital malformation.

In this imperfect world, the prospect of eliminating all of nature's baby-making errors may never be completely realized, but exciting advances in prenatal diagnosis are being made and applied today, as we shall see in the next chapter.

CHAPTER

VII

Windows on the Womb

By the time she was born, Susan Haynes possessed precious few secrets. She had been prodded, injected, chemically analyzed, electrocardiographed, and photographed both inside and out. Fortunately.

Susan was saved from death in the womb by intrauterine transfusion—an operation made necessary by the fact that her Rh-positive red blood cells were being destroyed by defensive antibodies from the Rh-negative blood of her mother. Susan was afflicted with Rh disease, erythroblastosis fetalis, which had killed the youngest of her three brothers shortly after birth.

Even more remarkable than the transfusion procedure, a ten-year-old miracle of the birth frontier, was the wide array of new diagnostic methods employed in Susan's case by doctors and technicians of Boston's Beth Israel Hospital, an affiliate of Harvard Medical School. They serve to illustrate the new kinds of tools and techniques that at last allow doctors to peer into the womb, to put the ill fetus within reach of rescuing hands.

"We were really conditioned to the idea that the baby probably would die," Susan's attractive, red-haired, thirty-four-year-old mother told me recently. (Susan's and her mother's name are changed in this account; all other details are authentic.) "It took a lot out of us . . . not knowing until the very end." Even with the array of sophisticated obstetrical techniques available at Beth Israel, the unborn Susan at best seemed to face a fifty-fifty chance for life.

But Mrs. Haynes's new obstetrician, Dr. Barry Schifrin, thirty-five, was encouraging. He explained that late in pregnancy he would inject red blood cells, matched to Mrs. Haynes's own blood, directly into the unborn baby, to replace the red blood cells destroyed by the antibodies.

The procedure is precarious for the unborn; on the average, one in twenty does not survive it. But at Beth Israel, special skills and equipment help to improve the odds.

The day before Mrs. Haynes's first intrauterine transfusion, she was wheeled into the hospital's ultrasonics laboratory. There, as a technician stroked her oiled, rounded abdomen with an ultrasonic wand, she was thrilled by her first glimpse of Susan—on a TV-like screen. "All you can see," says Mrs. Haynes, "are little lines and squiggles, but it's the outline of a little *body.*"

The ultrasonic picture showed just how Susan was lying in the womb, and the location of the placenta, which must not be penetrated by the needles used to inject dye or give the transfusion.

Dr. Schifrin injected a radiopaque dye into the amniotic fluid surrounding Susan. In the next twenty-four hours, Susan drank the fluid, which would end up in her gastrointestinal tract and outline it for the X ray as the target for the transfusion needle.

The next morning, given a sedative to quiet the baby so she would be a steady target, Susan's mother was wheeled into the fluoroscopy room and placed on an X-ray table where her abdomen was again bared, swabbed, and draped. As she watched, Dr. Schifrin deftly sank a four-inch hollow needle through her abdomen ("no more painful than a pinprick") into the uterus and amniotic sac. Following his progress by X ray, looking at the huge TV screen of the X-ray image intensifier, he kept advancing the hollow needle until it lodged and held in Susan's little abdominal cavity. He injected a bit of radiopaque dye into the cavity to verify his location; it registered on the TV screen. Then, through tubing that had been inserted through the needle, the concentrated blood—a lifesaving two to three ounces—was fed into Susan's body.

"It was marvelous," recalls Mrs. Haynes. "I watched it on television as they did it. You can see when they put the needle and the dye in, and the blood goes into the abdomen. I wasn't afraid."

Two weeks later, Dr. Schifrin administered another intrauterine transfusion. It went well. But the time was approaching, he decided, when Susan would be better off outside the womb, removed from her mother's damaging antibodies.

A sonic picture taken of Susan's head indicated a maturity of approximately thirty-six weeks, old enough for birth. Chemical tests of amniotic fluid were taken to verify the sonic reading.

Should the birth be induced? Could a distressed baby like this withstand the rigors of labor and normal delivery? Or must she be taken by Cesarean section, a major operation for the mother?

To find out, Dr. Schifrin performed a stress test. An ultrasonic device was placed on Mrs. Haynes's abdomen to monitor Susan's heartbeat in response to her mother's contractions, and record it on the graph of an electronic fetal monitoring machine beside her bed.

Mrs. Haynes was injected with oxytocin, a labor-stimulating drug—just enough to induce three fairly strong uterine contractions. During each contraction, Susan's heart remained stable—a normal pattern—and thus she passed the test. Otherwise, she would have been removed by Cesarean section that day.

A few days later, Mrs. Haynes met Dr. Schifrin promptly at 9 A.M. at Beth Israel Hospital for the birth of Susan. Soon she was in the labor room, attached to an intravenous line through which flowed labor stimulant. Two thin wires were inserted up the birth canal. One was attached to Susan's scalp to measure her pulse. Another, actually a thin plastic tube to measure pressure, floated free in the uterus. They connected to an electronic fetal monitor that recorded uterine contractions as well as Susan's heartbeat.

After six hours, the machine's tracings revealed that Susan was in trouble; the stress of the labor was beginning to show. A Cesarean section would be necessary after all.

Alerted to hazard by the ominous tracings, perinatologist Lawrence Minei and pediatrician Kishore Metha joined Dr. Schifrin and anesthesiologist Ivor Smith in the delivery room for the 4 P.M. Cesarean birth of Susan.

For an Rh baby, Susan was a big success. She was slightly blue in color, but breathing and vigorous, and weighed nearly five pounds. A few minutes later she was resting in the hospital's intensive-care nursery where she soon received another transfusion. Two weeks later she joined her mother and father and brothers at home.

These days, Susan, an energetic three-year-old, is a sturdy, happy playmate of her brothers, now nine and eleven.

"We wanted a sister for them," says Mrs. Haynes, smiling. "It was a chance we took."

One of the new obstetric methods used to diagnose Susan's condition was ultrasound. First it was employed to locate the baby and placenta, to safeguard the injection of dye. Then it measured the exact diameter of her head, as an indication of maturity. Finally, in the stress test, an ultrasonic device placed on the abdomen of Susan's mother monitored Susan's heartbeat.

But there are many other ways ultrasound is being employed to look in on the fetus. More than forty developmental disorders can be detected in utero by ultrasound. It can detect fetal life (or death), identify multiple pregnancies, chart growth (or warn of failure to grow, a bad sign). It aids the safe withdrawal of a sample of amniotic fluid. Obstetric diagnoses possible with ultrasound include blighted ovum, hydatidiform mole (a mass of cysts in the uterus), ectopic pregnancy (in which the embryo starts developing outside the uterus, a potentially fatal condition), placenta previa, hydrocephaly and anencephaly, hydramnios (excess amniotic fluid, potentially dangerous to the fetus), pregnancy complicated by myoma (a muscular tumor) or ovarian cyst.

Dr. Kenneth Gottesfeld, an obstetrician and a fetal ultrasonologist at the University of Colorado Medical Center, has seen fetal kidneys and even detected multiple cysts on the kidneys of one fetus, by means of ultrasound. He thinks it may be possible to determine fetal sex by observing on the scope the outlines of the genital region.

Obstetric ultrasound operates on the same principle used by the Navy to detect enemy submarines underwater, and by fishermen to locate schools of fish. Sound waves far above the limits of human hearing (2 million cycles per second versus 20,000 cps) are beamed toward the object to be detected. When they hit something they bounce back; the echoes are recorded as an echogram on an oscilloscope screen. A Polaroid picture of the screen is snapped if a permanent record is desired.

In many ways ultrasound does a better job than X ray, which poses a hazard to the fetus. (There has been no evidence that ultrasound as used is unsafe.) It shows up soft tissue structures that cannot be seen as well, or at all, by X ray, and does not require the injection into the subject of any substance, such as radiopaque fluid.

A different ultrasound method is known as the Doppler technique, used to record the fluctuations of a moving surface, such as a fetal heart or blood vessel. A Doppler transducer is placed on a woman's abdomen to pick up fetal heartbeat in electronic fetal monitoring.

Still another ultrasonic process known as time-motion display provides a continuous, shadowy moving picture of activity in the uterus. With it, reports a staff member of Montreal General Hospital, "We have seen twins fighting in the womb."

Dr. Fred Winsberg, a radiologist at Montreal General, has identified the fetal heart, aorta, intestinal loops, and the bladder, using motion-picture ultrasound. In connection with other types of ultrasound, in thirteen cases he has successfully estimated the blood output of the fetal heart from the left ventricle (thirty to forty drops of blood per heart stroke). And he believes that it is theoretically possible to detect congenital heart disease in the fetus with ultrasound, for this has already been done with newborns.

In the fast-moving, fast-growing field of ultrasonic diagnosis, advances are being made daily. Eventually, predicts Dr. Gottesfeld, ultrasonologists may be able to take a three-dimensional picture of the fetus and placenta, using ultrasonic holography. Few ultrasonic experts deny that great discoveries and wide applications of ultrasound lie ahead.

Another means of looking at the world of the fetus is more direct. Any time after the thirtieth week of gestation, some obstetricians now insert into the vagina a lighted endoscope, placing it up against the cervical membrane to view the color of the amniotic fluid. If the fluid is yellow-greenish rather than amber, it indicates that the fetus has passed meconium, the dark green secretion produced by fetal intestinal glands and normally excreted only after birth. This happens prenatally only during fetal distress, usually in times of oxygen deprivation, and is a sign that the fetus should be delivered. Up to one-third of all pregnancies need amniotic surveillance of this kind, according to one physician experienced in the technique, which is more popular in Europe than in the United States.

Dr. Carlo Valenti, professor of obstetrics at the State University of New York Downstate Medical Center, has directed development of a new kind of endoamnioscope good not only for peering, but for cutting, injecting, and cauterizing. With it, he has successfully visualized and taken tiny blood and flesh samples from fetuses in a score of pregnant women scheduled for hysterotomy (emptying of the uterus).

A telescopic fiberoptic lens is built into the small metal tube of the instrument, so that the physician can see the fetus. Other instruments that can be slipped into the tube include a needle for blood sampling or transfusion, a forceps for skin biopsy (sampling for analysis), and an electric cauterizing needle.

Dr. Valenti sees possible wide application for his new instrument, provided it proves safe for mothers and babies.

It can be used to diagnose fetal anatomical defects, such as spina bifida, and muscular disorders. Samples of fetal blood can be taken and analyzed for hereditary anemias such as sickle-cell disease, which could be detected in the tenth week of gestation—instead of at birth or later.

According to Dr. Valenti, the instrument would make it possible to transfuse blood safely into the fetus very early in pregnancy, under direct vision.

Faster predictions of fetal abnormalities would be another advantage. Cells from skin biopsies take only six to ten days to culture, as compared with twenty-five to thirty days to culture cells taken from amniotic fluid samples, which often do not hold enough viable cells for analysis. Thus a sample may be taken later in gestation, when there is less risk to the fetus, but still in time for therapeutic abortion should that prove necessary.

The endoamnioscope (also called the "uteroscope" or "fetuscope" by others) is not to be used casually, indicates Dr. Valenti, or in cases where other diagnostic techniques can serve as well. The thick, hollow probe cannot be inserted directly through the abdominal wall, as is the needle used for taking amniotic fluid samples. The abdomen must first be opened surgically. Then Dr. Valenti makes a tiny cut into the uterus, pushes the sharp point of the endoamnioscope through it and into the amniotic sac. After visually exploring whatever part of the fetus he wishes to examine, he inserts the biopsy instruments to cut and retrieve his sample. The puncture in the amniotic sac seals itself when the instrument is finally withdrawn.

Surprisingly, there was no bleeding in the biopsies initially taken by Dr. Valenti. "We speculate that the fetal intracapillary pressure must be lower than the pressure of the amniotic fluid," said Dr. Valenti. Thus the amniotic fluid acts as a seal to prevent bleeding from minor cuts, a fact that should ease the course of future fetal probes.

The amniotic fluid that surrounds the fetus is a protective buffer, the most intimate of many layers that long maintained the unborn as an untouchable mystery. Because it is so intimate to the fetus, the fluid he largely creates (part of the fluid is manufactured by the placental membranes), swims in, drinks, and excretes, it is now yielding up all kinds of secrets about him as an individual.

Amniocentesis is probably the most widely used and fruitful of all the new methods of fetal diagnosis. By means of a long hollow needle inserted through a pregnant woman's abdomen, a sample of amniotic fluid is drawn out for analysis.

There are several different kinds of things you can find out about a fetus by amniocentesis, points out obstetrician Allan C. Barnes, recently of Johns Hopkins University.

Sex of the fetus is the easiest determination to make. Skin cells sloughed off by the fetal body accumulate in the amniotic fluid; under the microscope all male cells are different from all female cells.

Where a fetus is likely to inherit a sex-linked disorder, such as hemophilia or muscular dystrophy (which affect only males), a decision to abort may hinge on a determination of fetal sex.

Age of the fetus is also indicated by discarded skin cells, suitably stained for easier analysis. The makeup of the skin changes week by week as the baby grows. Maturity of the fetal lungs can now be determined by measuring the ratio between lecithin and sphingomyelin in the amniotic fluid.

Physicians deciding whether to induce birth or perform a Cesarean section now depend heavily upon analysis of a teaspoonful of amniotic fluid. If delivered today, will the baby live? If not, what about seven days from now? Like generals mapping battlefield strategy, obstetricians in a high-risk perinatal center chart the probable outcome of a critical case. One line on the chart, reflecting chemical tests of fetal well-being, may indicate a buildup of toxins and probable death for the unborn baby within two and one-half weeks. A second line, sloping upward, shows increasing lung maturity and a good chance for life if the birth can be delayed ten days. So the mother may be put to bed, given oxygen, possibly sedated night and day with intravenous alcohol or nips of brandy; a dozen days later the baby is brought forth safely.

Chromosome count can be made by analysis of the discarded skin cells in the amniotic fluid—if enough live cells remain in the fluid sample. The live cells, cultured in little glass dishes, are grown for weeks in an incubator until there are enough of them for analysis. Usually ten to thirty cells are needed to make a diagnosis; each must be photographed under the microscope in the process of division; a drug is used to "freeze" them for the camera. The images of the cell chromosomes, forty-six to a normal cell, are cut out like jigsaw puzzle pieces and pasted up in line with the normal human chromosome arrangement. If the pieces do not quite fit, if some are missing or misplaced or added, certain types of defects can be diagnosed. Usually, any deviation from normal chromosome structure means that the child is gravely malformed—probably severely mentally retarded and also possibly badly handicapped physically.

About one birth in two hundred is affected by a chromosomal disorder.

Chemical composition of the amniotic fluid can be tested. This may reveal *metabolic disorders* caused by missing or defective enzymes, the catalysts that stimulate chemical reactions in the body. Generally, enzyme content in the amniotic fluid reveals any possible enzyme defect in the fetus. (Cultivated skin cells are also analyzed for this purpose.) Substances produced by metabolism may also be clues. Any one of some twenty-eight enzymes may be the reason for a metabolic disorder. Thus, a deficiency of one enzyme is believed to cause the digestive and respiratory difficulties of cystic fibrosis; lack of another makes it impossible for a baby to digest milk, a characteristic of galactosemia.

Bilirubin content of amniotic fluid is extremely useful in determining whether an Rh baby needs an intrauterine transfusion. A high level of bilirubin means that maternal antibodies are rapidly destroying the red blood cells of the fetus, causing severe anemia which if untreated could result in death. Or, if the fetus is sufficiently mature, birth may be induced to save him.

Gases dissolved in amniotic fluid can be measured. The gaseous tension of carbon dioxide in the amniotic fluid reveals the amount of oxygen the fetus is getting, and whether he is at risk.

Acidity of the amniotic fluid is also another indication of fetal distress, often caused by inadequate oxygen flow to the fetus.

More secrets of the amniotic fluid doubtless will be revealed before this book is published. Daily the study and practice of amniocentesis becomes more complex, more interesting to the specialist, more abstruse to the layman. Perhaps its human reality can best be grasped not by further technical descriptions but by examination of an actual case, one that happened last year in a small city in southern Wisconsin. Only the names of family members have been changed to protect their privacy.

A pregnancy at the age of forty-three can be worrisome. It was especially so for Mrs. Betty Thomas.

Not only was she at greater risk of a difficult pregnancy because of her age. Mrs. Thomas' big worry was that the unborn baby might carry the genetic defect of her first two children. Billy, born in 1949, who died seven months later, and Clark, born in 1952, were both afflicted with Down's sydrome, Mongolism, one of the chief genetic causes of mental retardation. It is in fact the source of 10 percent of all mental retardation.

Since that time Betty and her husband John had become parents of two normal daughters, now sixteen and eleven. Still the worry remained. Betty knew that the chances for anyone having a Mongoloid child increase with age. At age twenty, for the average mother, the chances are one in twenty-three hundred. From age forty to forty-five, that risk increases to one in one hundred (the risk of bearing a child with some kind of chomosomal abnormality at that age is one in forty). What were the odds for her?

As soon as he discovered she was pregnant, her family doctor referred Mrs. Thomas to Dr. Gloria Sarto, obstetrician and geneticist at the University of Wisconsin Medical School. In her laboratory in Madison, Dr. Sarto painlessly inserted a long needle through Mrs. Thomas' abdominal wall and into the amniotic sac to withdraw a sample of amniotic fluid.

Dr. Sarto took the small sample she obtained, concentrated the mixture by centrifuge, and then incubated the sample for weeks to allow the cells to multiply.

Generally, if a baby is normal, analysis shows forty-six normal chromosomes in each cell. But if the cells contain forty-seven chromosomes, caused by an extra small chromosome, the baby is a Mongoloid.

The test, combined with therapeutic abortion when indicated, can nearly ensure that no more Mongoloid children need be born to women so analyzed. (Most geneticists believe that pregnant women over forty should take the test, because of their higher risk of producing a Mongoloid child.) Similar procedures can be applied in the case of some fifty genetic disorders. Pregnancies with genetic defects can be aborted and normal pregnancies can take their places.

In states like Wisconsin where therapeutic abortions are forbidden after twenty weeks of pregnancy, the time factor is critical. To detect Mongolism, the amniotic fluid sample cannot be taken until the fourteenth week of pregnancy. Culturing and analyzing the sample takes four to six weeks, leaving only days before the twenty-week deadline for official approval of abortion and the procedure itself.

But good news came from Dr. Sarto in the sixth week. The geneticist was virtually certain that the unborn baby, a girl, was not a Mongoloid. However, analysis revealed, she was a carrier of the genetic defect, a chromosome rearrangement, and would have an increased risk of bearing children with Mongolism.

Tina Thomas, delivered a month early by Cesarean section, proved the accuracy of Dr. Sarto's forecast. Although small (four pounds, fifteen ounces) she was healthy and normal, bearing no traces of Down's syndrome. Finally Betty and John Thomas could shed the last vestiges of their worry.

A final chapter of the Thomas story is unfolding at this writing. Dr. Sarto has analyzed blood samples from Betty and John and found that Betty but not John carries the rearranged chromosome that increases the likelihood of having Mongoloid children. She now is analyzing blood samples from Betty's parents, to see if the defect goes back to them; if it does, blood samples from Betty's brothers and then perhaps their children (all normal) will need to be analyzed.

Blood analyses of the Thomas daughters, Jill, sixteen, and Joan, eleven, will reveal if they carry the trait. No matter what the finding, when they become mothers, modern genetics and obstetrics will help them to have normal babies.

CHAPTER

VIII

"I Had My Baby by Machine":
The Case for Fetal Monitoring

"The next time you have a baby," I asked Sally Hart, "would you want your doctor to use a monitor?"

"How can you ask a question like that?" came her immediate reply, "It saved my baby's life!"

But when Mrs. Hart, wife of a young lawyer, was first hooked up to an electronic fetal monitor, a large gray metal box with meters and oscilloscope and a blinking orange light, she was less than enthusiastic.

I'm perfectly normal, she thought. How could anything go wrong? It's pointless.

Most doctors would have agreed with her. Even if they are familiar with the electronic fetal monitor, available for general use only since 1969, the majority of obstetricians and family practitioners still regard it as a somewhat esoteric device, to be used only in pregnancies where the fetus is already ill or where difficult labor is expected.

Mrs. Hart's obstetrician, on the other hand, is one of a small, growing band of leading physicians who believe that eventually every birth will be guarded by an electronic monitor. They are sure that such monitoring can help greatly to reduce stillbirths, mental retardation, and neurological damage caused by the birth process. Such tragedies can happen even during the "normal" delivery, for one-third of problem babies are born to apparently healthy mothers.

Frequently, as in Sally's case, the trouble starts when the forces of labor pinch shut the umbilical cord, stopping the flow of life-giving blood to the baby. The effect of depriving the body and especially the brain of oxygen is identical to that of strangulation. It is the cause of nine out of ten cases of fetal distress and occurs in 25 percent of all births, though often the distress is brief and harmless.

Sally was a patient of Harvard Medical School's Dr. Barry Schifrin. When she went into labor, she checked into Boston's Beth Israel Hospital. There, despite some apprehension, she said nothing as a resident doctor painlessly inserted two wires from the monitor into her birth canal in less than a minute. One was clipped to the scalp of the unborn baby's head, lodged at the opening of the uterus. It would carry the baby's pulse, which would be registered as an electrocardiogram on the cathode screen; the heart rate would be plotted on the moving graph of the monitor. The second wire, actually a thin plastic tube, attached to a pressure sensor alongside the machine, continuously measured the frequency and strength of the uterine contractions. The relationship between these two lines on the graph enables obstetricians for the first time to tell what is really happening to a baby during labor and birth.

An hour later, at 11 A.M., recalls Sally, "Whoom! The pains became intense and frequent." When contractions came, Sally's husband Jim would coach her in the breathing patterns of the Lamaze method of prepared childbirth, which both had learned in classes at a hospital near Boston.

At 2:30 the heart rate pattern changed abruptly, and patterns thought to indicate significant umbilical cord compression began to appear on the graph.

The machine showed that at each contraction the baby's pulse would sink from 140 beats to 60 beats per minute or less. While changes in the baby's heart rate are common during labor, they are usually short-lived and return promptly to the previous rate. But the Smith baby's heartbeat recovered slowly, indicating that pressure against the umbilical cord was cutting off the baby's life-giving blood supply.

Cord compression is difficult or impossible to detect by the standard method of checking the fetal heartbeat with a stethoscope for thirty seconds every fifteen minutes—a method which monitors only 2 to 3 percent of the beats. Normally, explains Dr. Schifrin, the fetal heartbeat is not measured during a contraction. Not until continuous fetal monitoring was it possible for obstetricians to identify absolute patterns indicating that a cord was being pinched.

So began, recalls Sally, "three or four intense hours of 'sit up, lie down, move to here, move to there, lie on your side'" as nurses and doctors sought to shift the baby inside and prevent it from squeezing the umbilical cord that supported its life.

Each time Sally was moved or turned, the maneuver seemed to work. Watching the fetal monitor, doctors and nurses could tell that the blood supply was restored.

Without the monitor in this case, believes Dr. Schifrin, signs that the baby was being asphyxiated by a compressed cord could easily have been missed, with death or brain damage possibly the result.

Eventually the contractions became extremely long and more painful. While the baby's condition appeared stable, little progress in labor was evident.

Dr. Schifrin grew more discouraged, and began to consider doing a Cesarean section to remove the baby. However, at 7:08 P.M., Troy Hart, six pounds, nine and one-half ounces, came crying into the world—a bit blue but vigorous and apparently undamaged by the experience. A glance revealed the cause of his difficulties—the umbilical cord was wrapped in a figure 8 around his legs. At each contraction, his legs had been pressed together and had pinched the cord.

Relief and delight replaced anxieties. Dr. Schifrin, who had been hoarsely singing Christmas carols to ease the delivery room tension, broke into a chorus of "Jingle Bells," which mingled oddly with the cries of the Harts' new son.

It turned out that young Troy had weathered the storm beautifully. Today he is "playful and happy. He's a wonderful baby, completely healthy," I was told by Sally Hart, who won't mind a bit the next time she's attached to a fetal monitor.

A few weeks before the Hart birth, Dr. Schifrin had explained to me the reasons why he favors electronic fetal monitoring over standard obstetrical care. Dr. Schifrin, a former protégé of Dr. Edward H. Hon, the developer of electronic fetal monitoring, is a foremost investigator and consultant in the field.

"We're in a very interesting, very exciting time," Dr. Schifrin told me over coffee in his Boston office. "We're no longer at the behest of the fetus. We no longer believe that the fetus is the perfect parasite. Nor the perfect patient, paradoxically. He was for a while. He never complained very much. He suffered in silence. He came to the doctor only at the very last minute.

"It was believed that both the fetus and his environment were inviolable. You couldn't get to him. He was inscrutable.

"Fortunately and mercifully, we've given the lie to that. Babies can be reached, and they'd better be reached and understood if we're going to do anything about some very discouraging statistics."

Here Dr. Schifrin reached toward a pile of papers on his desk and withdrew an article from the *Journal of the American Medical Association* by a Dr. William F. Windle. "It is estimated," Dr. Schifrin read from the paper, "that there are no fewer than a half million victims of cerebral palsy and perhaps 6 million mental retardates in the United States. Once an hour an infant with cerebral palsy is being born; once every five minutes, one with mental retardation. The rate of crippling from these two is about 30 per 1,000 live births (one in 33). The cost to society is high. Just to provide institutional care for those most severely afflicted costs us well over a half billion dollars a year. We spend only a fraction of that for research on causes, treatment, and prevention."

Dr. Schifrin showed me the paper, which told how Dr. Windle had created cerebral palsy and mental retardation in just-born monkeys by duplicating conditions of fetal asphyxia. Asphyxiation for more than seven minutes invariably produced at least transient neurologic signs and permanent brain damage (revealed in autopsies).

"So a great deal of the brain damage we're talking

about could be prevented if only we knew . . ." I started to ask.

"Much of it, because we're beginning to relate much of it to asphyxia—especially the asphyxia that develops during labor and delivery. We don't think that all the problems relate to this. Some are caused by disease, for instance, and poor nutrition. But asphyxia at birth is very important.

"In addition to a pinched umbilical cord, asphyxia can be caused by a partially separated placenta that no longer feeds enough blood to the fetus; by pressure against the mother's inferior vena cava, which transports blood from the placenta and uterus to the heart; by prolonged contractions of the uterus, which prevent blood from getting from the placenta to the fetus; by drugs and anesthesia given the mother. These and other threats affect the fetal heart rate and thereby show up on the monitor.

"In addition to causing overt brain damage, we think asphyxia may result in minimal brain dysfunction, that may later show up as clumsiness, or behavior or reading problems. Roughly ten percent of babies who get to school have some degree of this. Or it may just knock ten or twenty points off one's IQ. Dr. Abraham Towbin has speculated that all of us might have a 'touch of mental retardation or other blight' as a result of slight brain damage sustained prenatally."

Can't standard obstetrical monitoring with a stethoscope reveal when a fetus is in trouble, in danger from asphyxia?

"The classical method of monitoring patients," replies Dr. Schifrin, "says that the safe range of fetal heart beat is one hundred and ten to one hundred and sixty beats per minute. Most doctors still believe that if you get outside either of these extremes, you've got fetal distress.

"Yet, a study of more than twenty-four thousand births by the Collaborative Project of the National Institute of Neurological Diseases and Stroke revealed virtually *no* correlation between fetal heart rate before birth and the condition of the baby delivered [as measured by the traditional intermittent monitoring by stethoscope]. A heart rate of sixty is not 'a step on the road to death' and a heart rate of one hundred and forty gives no assurance that a baby will be born in good condition.

"Increased irregularity in the heart rate is also considered a sign of fetal distress. But in fact in this NIH analysis no correlation was found.

"This study has not received the widespread publicity it deserves—not yet. But as our understanding of heart rate patterns from the fetal monitor increases, the less confidence we have in monitoring by stethoscope.

"Another interesting thing that was linked to this was the relationship of the people involved.

"If a group of obstetrical personnel seated in an auditorium are asked to count from a tape recorder representing fetal heart rate, you discover a very interesting thing—that obstetrical people count heart rates around one hundred forty beats per minute the best. The farther you go away from the normal range, the greater is the error in counting, and the greater is the tendency to correct.

"So—if you assume they listen a minute and a half in every half hour (three thirty-second listens), they're only listening five percent of the time. Also—they can't be relied on to count. . . .

"The biggest indictment of the auscultatory [listening] technique is that until the baby's delivered the obstetrician never knows which kind of baby he's going to face: one who is normal, one reversibly depressed, or one who is dead, dying, or retarded. This is indicated by the data from emergency Cesarean operations, performed in great haste to save the life of the baby. In most cases, the infant is found to be perfectly normal. The operation may have been unnecessary.

"What has happened is that obstetricians have come up with a bunch of magical numbers. For example, you leave a baby in utero for two hours if the mother is fully dilated—one hour if the mother has already had one child. Don't leave it in any longer because the incidence of trouble goes up with time. And if the heart rate goes down, you operate, because it has been firmly believed that low heart rate indicates approaching death—get the baby out before he dies.

"It is true that babies about to die have a lowered heart rate. But the contrary is not true—that all babies with a low heart rate are about to die.

"So the data has been totally unreliable.

"With electronic fetal monitoring, on the other hand, there's really enormous predictability. We've found that it's the *pattern* of heart rate that counts—not a heart rate sampled at an isolated moment in time. It's the pattern [measurable only with an electronic fetal monitor] and its relationship to uterine contractions. Each time the baby is squeezed the heartbeat changes in a characteristic curve.

"There's a belief among obstetricians that a baby can have a normal heart rate, say one hundred and forty when you listen, and ten minutes later the baby is dead. Yet it's never happened.

"We've seen babies who have had ominous patterns, babies who turned sour, but we've never seen a baby's heart just stop. In all the experience of fetal monitoring by major investigators, whereby we've had a continuous heart rate, there has never been an unexpected fetal death. To date, that involves twenty thousand to thirty thousand births.

"Our record of predicting a good fetal outcome approaches one hundred percent," said Dr. Schifrin, and here he showed me another paper from the pile on his desk—a March 6, 1972, article from the *Journal of the American Medical Association,* by Schifrin and Laureen Dame. "This study shows that if you take a group of babies who have normal heart patterns, as shown by the electronic fetal monitor, they have normal outcomes, and if you take a group of babies with ominous heart rate patterns, there are a number of babies who do poorly (none of the babies with correctable problems was included in the study). We analyzed the patterns blindly—we just read the graphs emitted by the monitors, with no other information on these three hundred and seven births."

If the fetal monitor signals trouble, what happens next? Repositioning of the mother, as happened with Sally Hart; oxygen and possibly intravenous fluids given to the mother; and, as a last resort, a Cesarean section performed in a few minutes. A rule of thumb is that if an ominous pattern in a previously healthy baby cannot be corrected with half an hour, it's time to operate.

Proof is accumulating that electronic monitoring combined with these measures really works. At Los Angeles County–University of Southern California Medical Center, for example, one-fourth of all patients are monitored—those believed by the physicians to be high risk. These would be expected to have twice as many stillbirths as those in the normal group. In fact, apparently because they are monitored, they have *half* as many fetal deaths during labor and delivery as the low-risk group, one-fourth the expected number.

It is estimated that 40 percent of all stillbirths in this

country occur after labor begins, that each year 28,000 apparently normal babies die in the process of being born. Could fetal monitoring also cut this rate by three-fourths?

Use of the fetal monitor prevents unnecessary Cesarean sections, as in the case of Sally Hart. Fetal monitoring can be used to modulate the effect of medication and pain-relieving agents which frequently cause asphyxia in the unborn baby. A pioneering study done by Dr. Schifrin revealed that when oxytocin (a stimulant used worldwide to induce births) was given to women in labor, 25 percent of all fetuses showed asphyxiation patterns. When epidural anesthesia (the least severe regional anesthesia) was used, 20 percent of fetuses evoked such patterns (some only moderate, some severe). But when oxytocin and anesthesia were used together, 50 percent of all unborn babies showed asphyxiation patterns.

If the electronic monitor is employed, the physician can note dangerous patterns and correct medication so that episodes of asphyxia are transient, not harmful. "We have been able to drastically reduce these patterns," says Dr. Schifrin, "by maintaining patients on their side during labor, and controlling the rate of oxytocin infusion with a constant infusion pump."

A monitor makes better use of doctors' and nurses' time—and makes sure they are there when most needed. (One person at a central console with duplicate screens can follow all labors simultaneously.) It focuses attention on the patient most at risk—the baby.

Fetal monitoring can prevent the element of surprise. If a fetus is in trouble, there is time to call a pediatrician to be on hand to resuscitate the baby at delivery if necessary. Or an ambulance can be sent from a regional newborn intensive-care center to take the baby to more sophisticated staff and facilities.

Electronic monitoring can extend the reach of consultants. Dr. Schifrin, for example, receives fetal monitoring patterns transmitted by telephone line from Waltham Hospital ten miles away, and helps interpret the tracings. Dr. Gerald G. Anderson, at Yale, has set up a similar service, twenty-four hours a day, that is planned eventually to reach every hospital maternity ward in Connecticut.

The machine is an important follow-up and research tool even after birth. The complete electronic fetal monitoring record of each birth is preserved on paper and can be filed with other records. Years later, it can help investigators in comparing the effectiveness of different kinds of obstetric techniques in averting brain damage. And the monitor can be invaluable in testing the safety of new medications given mother or fetus.

Electronic fetal monitoring is now being introduced widely across the United States. More than 10 percent of the 5200 hospital maternity wards in the United States have electronic fetal monitoring equipment, but few are fully equipped. Usually, a hospital has a single unit capable of monitoring one labor at a time. Most major manufacturers of medical monitoring equipment produce a fetal monitor.

A new feature now available is an external ultrasonic sensor to detect the fetal heartbeat. There is also an external device, a belt with a strain gauge that fits around the laboring woman to record labor contractions. So a nurse can apply both before the doctor comes.

Various companies and universities—including Yale, Harvard, U.S.C., and the universities of Wisconsin and Alabama—are working on a computer-controlled system that can read a tracing and sound a warning when the baby is in trouble.

With all of these advantages, why isn't electronic fetal monitoring universally employed? Why do many brand-new machines sit unused on hospital shelves while women in labor go unmonitored? I asked Barry Schifrin.

"For one thing, obstetricians think that this new method is very complex, hard to understand. It isn't. If any medical group runs fearfully, it's the obstetricians. They have the mother *and* the baby to handle. And while it's very appropriate that they be very conservative about accepting new techniques, this has limited their acceptance of the limitations of the techniques they now use.

"There's another thing. An obstetrician thinks: 'If a birth I manage is monitored and I do something wrong, the evidence may be there on the graph. Am I liable for suit?' So he's not going to monitor until the laws change and it's grounds for malpractice not to monitor."

Will it be grounds for a malpractice suit someday not to monitor a birth?"

"Well, yes, when monitoring takes its place in the standard care of obstetric cases, which I am sure will happen. Would it be malpractice for a cardiologist not to use an electrocardiograph? I think so. What part of cardiology is an electrocardiograph? Not a hell of a lot. It just tells you whether or not the patient has a problem.

"Electronic fetal monitoring is only a small part of obstetrics. But right now it's revolutionary. And the impact that this technique is going to have on obstetrics will be enormous."

Wide adoption of this new system, as with any new procedure, cannot be immediate nor entirely easy.

The electronic fetal monitor is not a magic box that all by itself is going to save lives or prevent brain damage.

Like any new piece of medical equipment, it needs to be operated by people who know how to use it and how to take care of it. Otherwise it is a failure.

It is not a device to save the doctor's time—in fact, it increases the demand for skilled medical or paramedical attention. The information it presents continuously isn't of any use unless someone looks at it, and then is prepared to do something if an ominous pattern develops. Its development emphasizes the need, stressed by the American College of Obstetricians and Gynecologists, for consolidation of obstetrical wards into fewer, larger, more sophisticated centers which can afford expensive equipment and highly trained staffs. Nurses and technicians must be trained to read and interpret electronic fetal monitors; doctors alone will not have the time.

Cost is a factor. Each monitor at this writing costs about $5000. But the life of a monitor is easily five years; if it is used on only two hundred births a year the amortization is only $6 per patient and disposable supplies are no more than $10. Some hospitals simply add a $25 charge to the patient's bill for monitoring, which is paid for by some Blue Cross and other health insurance policies.

Does the monitor frighten the patient or dehumanize the birth process? There is a tendency, some say, for nurses to sit and watch the monitor screen and forget the patient. But, says Dr. L. Stanley James, Columbia University neonatologist, "the development of modern technology doesn't necessarily mean an exclusion of a warm, human, understanding environment. People are surrounded in their homes by various electric and electronic appliances, such as the TV. When they come to the hospital, they expect to have new forms of instrumentation. If you can explain to the mother that you are just getting more information as to how the baby is doing, she is delighted to have it."

One obstetrician reports that his patients who have been monitored once insist that in the future "I want to have my babies by machine!"

Says James: "I think we will eventually come to the stage where if we are going to manage patients correctly we are going to monitor them all. Most won't be with a clip on the baby's scalp, but with external monitoring devices that are completely convenient, comfortable, smaller, handier, and lower in cost."

Dr. James, who is chairman of the American Academy of Pediatrics' Committee on the Fetus and the Newborn, talked with me of the next stage in fetal monitoring—computerization.

"Here at Columbia–Presbyterian Hospital we've just begun a two-year, hundred-thousand-dollar program to apply computer technology to monitoring in labor. I think computerization is going to have a really great impact on obstetrics and newborn care.

"Of course, the computer is just a big adding machine; it doesn't make any diagnoses. But it can add and sort information useful to the obstetrician and nursing staff. For example, you might ask the computer to summarize the last eight hours of uterine contractions—their strength and frequency and their probable effect on the baby. This would give precise information, say, to a new shift of maternity nurses coming on duty."

A few months later and a continent away, I talked with the world's leading authority on electronic fetal monitoring, about computerization and the future of monitoring.

The name of Dr. Edward H. Hon, an engineer and professor of obstetrics and gynecology, University of Southern California, is synonymous with electronic fetal monitoring. Beginning at Yale Medical School in 1959, he led the development of fetal monitoring techniques and equipment. By studying patterns from thousands of births, he has developed means of interpreting them and has compiled an atlas of normal and abnormal patterns that is the definitive book in the field. Since 1969, in company with Dr. Edward J. Quilligan, former chief of obstetrics at Yale, Dr. Richard Paul, former research fellow at Yale, and other outstanding specialists including biomedical and electronics engineers, he has continued his investigations at the Los Angeles County–University of Southern California Medical Center. The huge hospital serves an indigent population of 1.5 million—70 percent Mexican and Mexican-American—in east Los Angeles, and delivers 10,000 babies per year. Some 3000 of these births—to women considered high risk—are monitored electronically.

"Will computers soon be used to help monitor patients?" I asked Dr. Hon.

"Yes," he said. "We think one of the great problems in monitoring at present is that great masses of data accumulate even during a ten-hour labor. There's a lot of material for the doctor to digest. We're in the process here of developing a computing fetal monitor that does a lot of measurements for the doctor and presents these in numerical form. In fact the plans for it are all worked out and I expect to have a prototype model soon. It won't be costly, so it will be within reach of all hospitals that now use monitors.

"The system will use present fetal monitors. To each monitor we'll add a black box that will do the computing. The black box will compute the fetal risk index of the patient. This would be a composite index —a number—that would take into consideration the clinical history of the patient, the things that are going on during this particular labor. If the index is rising, it means the baby is endangered, so you'd better do something. If the index is steady or falling, you can be very confident of a good outcome. This index number (in our present plan) would be updated every ten minutes, so you would get a running report on your baby.

"A minicomputer at a central point will oversee all the monitors in the hospital. There will be a keyboard in which we will punch in the clinical history of the patient, and there will be a printing terminal. There will also be a large display board that will list all patients in labor. If a patient is having trouble, her name will start flashing on and off. The doctor punches a button and gets a printout of the patient's clinical history. He punches another button and gets a data sheet summarizing all the things that happened during the course of labor on this patient, including a complete running record of fetal index numbers calculated at ten-minute intervals."

A few minutes later I was standing with Dr. Roger Freeman in U.S.C.'s research delivery room, where new forms and programs of monitoring are tested. Here, each day, one especially difficult or interesting birth is studied. The delivery room itself is standard, but behind a large picture window is a room banked with computers, with monitors and data processing equipment. Here, already, computers are cooperating with obstetricians to make births safer.

Not only the fetus but the mother is monitored electronically, explained Dr. Freeman, for heart rate and also blood pressure. Results are visualized by oscilloscope and printed readouts; through use of the computer, findings are compared with diagnostic standards. Blood samples may be taken from the scalp of the unborn baby and analyzed for acidity, which builds up if the fetus is deprived of sufficient oxygen. ("Fetal blood sampling is awkward, it's inconvenient, and you can't do it quite as early as you can monitor the fetal heart," Dr. Hon had said. "I think generally around the world today most people would believe that what you do is monitor the heart rate and if you find funny changes in it that you don't understand, then you get a fetal blood sample. Even Saling, who developed the blood-sampling technique, believes that.") In this research installation, physicians study such things as the relationship between fetal heart rate and blood acidity, the effect on the fetus of maternal anesthesia, the response to oxytocin challenge tests, and the value of various types of treatment. "What we have learned here," wrote Dr. Edward Quilligan in *Hospital Practice*, "has considerably improved practice throughout the obstetric clinical department."

One of the most important new indices being tested in the research delivery room, explained Dr. Freeman, is the beat-to-beat difference in fetal heart rate. In the normal heartbeat, each interval between beats is a little shorter or longer than the next, with a maximum difference of 0.025 seconds between beats, and three to five similar cycles per minute. "As long as the central nervous system is controlling the heart, you get these little differences all the time. But if your brainstem were cut off, your heart rate would be perfectly smooth. There would be no variation from one beat to the next. The important thing is that we can look at central nervous system control of the heart through the beat-to-beat difference. We can see the effects of drugs on the beat-to-beat rate, for example, long before we see them in the actual speeding up or slowing down of the heart. Prematurity, toxemia, and fetal oxygen starvation may eliminate the beat-to-beat difference, which may well be an ominous sign. But we'll be able to act faster."

Later, talking again with Dr. Hon in his office, I asked about changes expected in monitoring the fetus weeks before birth.

"That's an area that needs developing," he said. "There will be more of that, as in the present oxytocin challenge test. All of our effort has been directed at the labor period. But now we're moving backward toward conception, and we're in the process of building better equipment to get information on the younger fetus. So that will be a whole new area of expansion, and the other area is newborn monitoring. There is as yet no real body of information on the newborn heart rate and respiration such as we have on the fetal heart rate.

"The wide-spectrum kind of monitoring we've been doing in the fetus is only just beginning to be done on the newborn."

"And isn't being done in adults at all?" I asked.

"No," said Dr. Hon, his eyes twinkling with anticipation. "There's another fascinating area. The beat-to-beat difference in heart rate. This is not being used at all today by the cardiologists, and the possibilities are exciting."

In its infancy, electronic fetal monitoring appears destined to grow and grow.

CHAPTER

IX

Newborn Rescue

Birth almost always is normal, healthy, happy. The typical newborn is fit and tough, even if born of a high-risk mother. And thirty-two out of thirty-three newborns can be cared for perfectly well in the average hospital nursery, or at home.

This chapter is all about the one baby in thirty-three who needs ultraspecial care to survive—a type of care that was unavailable in America only a few years ago, and is provided today in less than two hundred Newborn Intensive-Care Units (NICUs) scattered across the continent. More NICUs are needed.

Amid scenes reminiscent of the "baby hatcheries" of science-fiction movies, a new breed of doctors and nurses works around the clock to save the lives of the tiniest humans. Constantly developing and testing new theories, changing and improving techniques and equipment, they are making advances that ultimately will benefit all babies everywhere.

Scott seemed normal at birth, except that when he cried, his skin turned blue-black. His worried doctor, suspecting oxygen lack due to a heart malformation, telephoned for help. In three hours, a small red plane had landed on the little airstrip near Scott's hometown of Afton, Wyoming. It carried a doctor-nurse team who tucked Scott carefully into a portable incubator and fed him oxygen as the wind-buffeted aircraft bore them 140 miles back to Salt Lake City, Utah.

There, at the Intermountain Newborn Intensive Care Center of the University of Utah Medical Center, X rays revealed the exact nature of the birth defect Scott's doctor had suspected. A pediatric heart surgeon made a new opening in the tiny heart to attain a normal blood flow and ended the threat to Scott's life.

Such rescues happen daily in the dramatic world of newborn intensive care. Eskimo infants, some who weigh a scant two pounds, frequently are airlifted 1500 miles from Baffin Island to Montreal Children's Hospital. Helicopters transport ill and premature babies from all over Maryland to a Baltimore NICU, and from central California and western Nevada to Stanford University Hospital.

Within ten minutes after receiving a call regarding an ill infant from any point within a hundred-mile radius, a specially equipped ambulance zooms away from the University of Michigan's NICU at Ann Arbor. Aboard, with a prewarmed portable infant incubator containing its own oxygen, heat, and power supply, are a pediatrician, a registered nurse, and a respiratory therapist.

In San Francisco; Pensacola, Florida; and New York City, a large van equipped as a mobile intensive-care nursery rolls to the rescue. Better equipped than many small hospital nurseries, with such things as incubators, monitors, and resuscitators, a minilaboratory, treatment fluids and medications, with full facilities for massive blood transfusions or minor surgery, the units are manned by doctors and nurses experienced in infant rescue techniques.

Ideally, a baby expected to need intensive care is transported to a high-risk center *before birth* in the best possible incubator—his mother's body. He is delivered across the street or better yet across a corridor from a newborn intensive-care unit.

Even then, like Jimmy, he may face extraordinary hazards.

When Jimmy was born, two months premature, he took one gasp and stopped breathing. His body was limp, and turning blue from lack of oxygen. Moving quickly, a pediatrician used a tiny vacuum pipe to suction mucus from his throat and breathing passages, then inserted another tube down his windpipe. At the other end was a rubber bag filled with oxygen-rich air, which the pediatrician pumped rhythmically to begin the process of breathing.

In the intensive-care nursery next door, alerted nurses had prepared a plastic-topped incubator to receive Jimmy. Like an artificial womb, it and its attachments would furnish him with basic needs during the next critical hours and days: oxygen, warmth, fluids. As Jimmy was placed within its embrace, a nurse fitted a respirator mask over his face; a machine began to help him breathe.

The pediatrician inserted a catheter in Jimmy's umbilical artery; it would remain, like an artificial umbilical cord, to be used for drawing blood samples, especially to ascertain the oxygen level in Jimmy's blood so it could be maintained at a precise level. Too little oxygen could result in irreparable damage to Jimmy's brain, causing some degree of mental retardation,

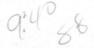

cerebral palsy, or even death. Too much oxygen over too long a time could damage the retina in his eyes.

But little Jimmy rapidly began to improve. Within twenty-four hours he was breathing for himself; his pulse and color were good and he was well on the way to a completely healthy life.

Newborn intensive care is not only expected by experts to cut U.S. infant mortality in half. Far more important is its effect on the quality of babies saved.

Less than a generation ago, it was not believed possible to *prevent* mental retardation and neurological defects. The causes were largely unknown, and often ascribed simply to heredity.

Then investigators began to discover a shocking truth: while many cases of brain damage were caused by genetic or chromosomal defects, by insults to a baby's brain in the womb or during birth, others developed *in the hospital nursery*, frequently in the first few hours of life. With better efforts to detect and correct deficiencies or complications, many babies could be saved from lifelong mental disability.

So began the pediatric subspecialty known as neonatology. Neonatologists—pediatricians with advanced training or experience in this field—began careers devoted to medical care in the newborn period, usually considered to be the first twenty-eight days of life, and to learning more about the prenatal development of the baby. They evolved new techniques and Lilliputian equipment especially suited to their tiny patients.

By 1967, with initial Federal help, a handful of NICUs under the direction of neonatologists were in operation—at such places as the medical centers of Yale, Columbia, Western Reserve, Vanderbilt, Baylor, the University of California, and Stanford. Today, virtually all major medical centers contain such a unit.

"Probably no area of medicine has witnessed such tremendous changes as has care of the newborn infant," declares Dr. L. Stanley James.

Unlike the standard hospital nursery, which may allot ten babies to a nurse, a typical NICU maintains a ratio of two babies to a nurse in the newcomer ward, three to one in the intermediate area, and four or five to one in the "graduate" section. In certain cases, one nurse will be assigned to care for just one baby.

The staff is aided by space-age equipment unknown only a few years ago, including:

A mechanism that continuously measures the baby's skin temperature and adjusts the heat of the incubator accordingly.

Sensors attached to the baby that monitor heartbeat, breathing, and blood pressure, and that sound alarms and blink lights to warn of danger.

Oxygen analyzers and regulators to keep oxygen intake at prescribed levels.

Infusion pumps that drip intravenous fluids containing glucose, water, salts, proteins, and sometimes antibiotics into a baby's bloodstream at a preset rate through a catheter inserted in his umbilical artery.

Blood samples may be taken many times around the clock and each analyzed within a few minutes. Intravenous fluids and oxygen levels are changed accordingly to preserve a fragile life.

Blood is always on hand for minute transfusions— as little as half an ounce for a five-pound baby, which is the equivalent of a pint of blood given a 160-pound adult.

Always on call for consultation is the neonatologist who directs the NICU; at times he may stay for hours at the side of a critically ill newborn. And on the spot night and day are a resident M.D., a chief nurse, and perhaps a certified pediatrician, a "Fellow" in training to become a neonatologist.

Near at hand in the ideal medical center are pediatric subspecialists available nowhere else in the area— an anesthesiologist, a cardiologist, a gastroenterologist, a neurologist, and others whose sole practice is concerned with the peculiarities of children's diseases. Frequently such consultants are located in a pediatric hospital, such as Children's Memorial in Chicago, or Toronto's Hospital for Sick Children.

By far the largest number of babies in an NICU are premature; three pounds is a common weight. And by far the majority of prematures are victims of breathing difficulty, because their lungs are immature.

Twins Danny and Andrea were examples of immaturity and respiratory distress, the twin problems that together or separately account for 75 percent of all newborn deaths. Born eight weeks prematurely, each weighed about three pounds. Danny appeared to be stillborn, and doctors weren't even sure he had a pulse, but efficient resuscitation saved his life. Both babies were placed in their own monitored incubators filled at first with nearly 100-percent oxygen.

Still, as happens to some degree in all babies with severe respiratory distress, the dread hyaline membrane began to coat the linings of their lungs' tiny alveoli (air sacs) and bronchioles (minute branches of the bronchial tubes). Related to the immaturity of the lungs of prematures, aggravated by chilling or other stress, hyaline membrane disease—also known as respiratory distress syndrome (RDS)—accounts for half of all newborn deaths.

The twins were born before their lungs started to manufacture sufficient surfactant. Without the fluid, the air sacs collapse at each breath like brand-new toy balloons. Each breath is an effort for the baby; he grunts or moans; his nostrils flare, and without additional oxygen he begins to turn blue.

Andrea was treated with a recently developed technique—continuous positive airway pressure (CPAP) —that has dramatically increased the chances of RDS-afflicted babies. Developed by University of California pediatric anesthesiologist Dr. John Gregory, it involves propping open the air sacs at all times by application of a constant low pressure to the lungs. This may be done by various means. For Andrea, it was through a tube inserted down her windpipe. For a baby nearby, it was by means of a close-fitting pressurized hood around the head, with oxygen-rich, humidified air being pumped in and out. Dr. Victor Chernik in Winnipeg, Manitoba, has achieved the same result by placing a vacuum or negative-pressure hood around the baby's chest—it creates a "weightless" or lifting effect; as in other CPAP techniques, the lungs are not allowed to exhale fully. And at Western Reserve University's NICU, RDS newborns are benefiting from a discovery that eliminates the need for an endotracheal tube (a tube that fits into the windpipe). Air is fed through carefully fitted nostril plugs; since babies are compulsive nose breathers, air does not escape through the mouth and the pressure is maintained.

The CPAP technique not only makes the lungs more efficient, breathing easier, and the heart strain less, but it also allows for a sharp decrease in the concentration of oxygen, which can damage lungs as well as eyes.

CPAP is not for all RDS babies; it is not for tiny babies like Danny who did not breathe spontaneously at birth. He was treated with a different respiratory technique.

Because of his cramped condition before birth,

Danny was born with a concave chest. Every time he exhaled his chest would collapse. To counter this, and also because of his general weakness, he was attached to a respirator that breathed for him. Tubes led through his nostrils down to his lungs, supplying a monitored, humidified air-oxygen mixture under alternating pressure.

As soon as he could breathe on his own, the respirator was removed so he would not become dependent upon it. Andrea too was soon able to give up her breathing equipment.

Gradually the oxygen level given the twins was lowered; as usually happens with RDS babies, by the time Danny and Andrea were a few days old, their lungs were manufacturing sufficient surfactant; they were over the RDS crisis. But other fearsome problems developed.

Andrea had an immature heart that at times would slow from a normal rate of 140 beats per minute down to a complete halt. But taped to her chest was an electrode that picked up her heartbeat. It was wired to a monitor that emitted a warning electronic squeal when the heartbeat slowed. In seconds an alerted nurse would reach into the isolette to shake Andrea's arm or leg.

Usually this simple stimulation is enough to speed up a newborn's heart or start him breathing. It's needed so frequently that some babies are equipped with a nurses' invention known as a "hey-you!" stick —a tongue depressor attached by gauze to a baby's leg. A pull on the string jerks the leg and startles the immature neurological system, reminding it to keep heart and lungs pumping. If that doesn't work, one nurse restarts breathing with a bellows attached to a face mask, while another administers external heart massage, rhythmically depressing the baby's tiny breastbone with her two fingers.

Danny and Andrea next faced the onslaught of jaundice—a condition that develops in most premature babies. Their immature livers cannot efficiently excrete a normal waste, bilirubin, which is so toxic it can damage brain tissue if allowed to build up in the blood.

Continuous phototherapy for many hours cleared up the jaundice; otherwise blood transfusions would have been necessary. Phototherapy, in use for more than a decade, involves exposing the naked infant (eyes covered) to bright fluorescent light similar to daylight. The light penetrates the baby's skin and causes a breakdown of bilirubin into harmless chemicals.

The twins did so well that they were deemed out of danger in two weeks and released from the intensive-care unit to the regular hospital nursery. They were home with their parents in another six weeks. And by the time they were brought back for a checkup at age six months, they were fat and healthy. Andrea had grown to fourteen and one-half pounds, Danny to sixteen and one-half. Whether either had neurological damage would be checked on in future examinations; NICU graduates are usually observed for five years.

A minor although important threat to the very young are infectious diseases, accounting for about 5 percent of newborn deaths. Most dangerous is septicemia, a generalized infection of the blood that is treated with antibiotics. Another frequent infection is pneumonia, the affliction of Margarita—brought in from another nursery and placed in an incubator marked ISOLATION.

"Most physicians know how to handle infection and

fight it with antibiotics," explains a neonatologist. "The problem is that the baby is so sick he requires the constant surveillance by and constant availability of physician and nurse, plus monitoring equipment. And this is normally only available in an intensive-care unit."

(Most infections don't spread easily through the air, a fact which makes it possible to group ill newborns in NICUs. Furthermore, air introduced into the incubators is filtered, and some NICUs are equipped with special air-flow systems designed to spirit contaminants away quickly. Scrupulous hand washing with antiseptics by anyone handling babies, and similar precautions, cut down the spread of germs.)

Birth trauma—such as rare cerebral hemorrhage caused by pressure upon the head during difficult delivery—accounts for another 5 percent or so of infant deaths.

Congenital malformations, such as the heart defect Scott was born with, cause 10 percent of newborn deaths. Malformations may be caused by infections contracted before birth, by certain chemicals, drugs or radiation during the prenatal period, by inheritance or simply by a mistake of nature in forming the developing embryo.

Also, babies of diabetic mothers frequently end up in intensive care. Typically, Kit was premature but larger than most full-term babies. When he was a fetus, his mother's elevated blood sugar had affected him: it caused his pancreas to produce large amounts of insulin, which not only reacted with the sugar but acted on his body as a growth stimulant. (Insulin is a protein hormone.) Because he was large, his birth was difficult and slow, posing the threat of asphyxia.

When Kit was born, his overactive pancreas for a time kept producing excess insulin, which rapidly eliminated his own blood sugar. NICU doctors expected the low blood sugar condition, and tested it quickly and simply by analyzing drops of blood taken from his heel. They treated it by intravenous feeding of glucose, together with calcium to elevate that mineral to its normal level in his blood. At one point sodium bicarbonate was added when the blood became too acid.

Because Kit was immature, his lungs developed hyaline membrane disease, a mild case that rapidly improved under the administration of high levels of oxygen. Frequent blood-gas tests guarded against the possibility of oxygen overdosage.

Jumping one disease hurdle after another in quick succession, Kit was pink and healthy just two and one-half weeks after his birth, when he was sent home with his parents.

A newborn intensive-care unit is ever a place of high drama. At any moment a brand-new baby is fighting to retain his life. Another, perhaps watched by parents, obviously is losing his. A third wavers on the edge, his odds changing by the hour. Around each baby like robot sentinels stands elaborate life-support equipment, respirators tapping with each breath, oscilloscopes greenly marking the progress of each heartbeat.

What kind of a nurse can work in such an atmosphere?

"It helps to carry a screwdriver," says one. "With all this equipment, you need to develop a mechanical sense."

"Her interest in those babies is the most important thing," says an NICU chief of nurses. "And to function in this tense place she has to be emotionally stable."

An RN or an LPN (Licensed Practical Nurse), she

needs at least nine months of additional in-service training before handling all aspects of nursing care. Frequent lectures by various medical center department chiefs instill theory and techniques.

But cold efficiency is not enough. Nurses in the best NICUs are encouraged to love their patients, to coo to and cuddle them, to provide the social and emotional stimulation they need in order to thrive.

At many NICUs, including those of the University of Wisconsin, Western Reserve University, and University of California, San Diego, parents and grandparents are encouraged to visit their babies in the nursery any time of the day or night, to touch and fondle and feed them. Mothers are allowed to breastfeed, if at all feasible.

At some NICUs, physicians, interns, and medical students are encouraged to walk through the nursery whenever they care to. They don't even need to don a mask or gown (unless they handle a baby). "The more medical people who help us observe our babies, the better," explains a neonatologist who follows the open nursery policy. The practice gained popularity after a pioneering 1968 study at Columbia–Presbyterian Babies Hospital in New York, which showed *lower* mortality and less major bacterial infection during open periods.

How successful are NICUs?

Infant death rates usually drop dramatically when a region opens a newborn intensive-care unit. In its first year of operation, the NICU at the University of Tennessee cut mortality among premature babies by 25 percent. The University of Mississippi NICU halved the death rate for prematures weighing at least 3.3 pounds. Metropolitan Toronto, served since 1960 by the outstanding NICU at the Hospital for Sick

Children, experienced a drop in overall newborn mortality (deaths during the first twenty-eight days of life) from 15.4 per thousand live births in 1961 to 10.1 in 1971.

In 1970, neonatologist Joan E. Hodgman, M.D., established an NICU at Los Angeles County Medical Center, which serves only indigents. By 1972, the newborn death rate at the hospital had plunged from 18.2 per thousand live births to 12.2. (Lower, in this poor population, than the national average in 1972 of 13.8.) Mortality for babies weighing more than five and one-half pounds at birth sank from over 0.4 percent to 0.2 percent.

But what about the quality of the lives saved? Are the babies who would have died now living crippled or retarded?

"It is sometimes argued," says a recent monograph of the Ontario Council of Health, *Perinatal Problems*, "that a reduction in perinatal deaths by proper reproductive care would result in an increased number of permanently handicapped individuals. The opinion is based upon studies carried out before the recent revolutionary changes in perinatal care. . . .

"The evidence is now beginning to accumulate that such assumptions regarding inevitable morbidity are no longer justified. Thus, a recent study shows that 86.7 percent of 72 infants surviving a birth weight of less than 1,500 grams [3.3 pounds] are apparently normal and only 7.4 percent definitely abnormal. Survivors of artificial ventilation have a normal distribution of I.Q. compared with controls. . . ."

Furthermore, suggests the publication, NICU care would actually reduce the total number of mentally retarded and neurologically damaged individuals who are added to society each year. For "measures that prevent death may also prevent brain damage (in those who would survive even standard care), as for example in the prompt and correct treatment of neonatal asphyxia, jaundice, and hypoglycemia [low blood sugar]."

Genetic counseling, family planning, antenatal diagnosis, selective therapeutic abortion, and fetal and maternal monitoring in labor undoubtedly could further lower the production of mental defectives.

Dr. Edward J. Quilligan of U.S.C. has estimated that the cost to the community of lifetime medical and custodial care for an individual, brain damaged at birth, is $500,000. Thus, concludes the Ontario report, "the estimated costs of treatment for the high-risk delivery at $2,500 and for an infant in a neonatal intensive care unit at $3,200 are relatively low."

What of the future of newborn intensive care?

"The whole field of intensive care is really in its infancy," says Columbia's L. Stanley James. "With new technology, new techniques, new knowledge at hand, there are going to be vast changes. We haven't even begun to arrive at the full potential."

Among the latest examples of advanced technology:

A tape, applied to an infant's skin, that changes color to reflect changes in the baby's temperature.

A special air mattress that triggers an alarm if the baby resting on it stops breathing.

A cigarette-sized electronic probe, inserted beneath the skin, that measures blood acidity.

A tiny electrode, inserted through a catheter into a newborn's aorta to monitor blood gas continuously and prevent harmful oxygen concentrations.

"We must streamline and miniaturize our instrumentation," says Dr. James, who is consulted frequently by designers of new NICU equipment. "The incubator itself, which has made a great contribution in isolating the infant from infection, maintaining him in a stable environment, will be redesigned completely to permit easy access to the baby in an emergency. All of the various life-support accessories, such as intravenous pumps, blood pressure monitors, oxygen, suction, respirator, get in the way of care and make it hard to move the baby, as when he is taken to surgery or X ray. The new incubator will incorporate these accessories into its design so that it becomes a kind of self-contained intensive-care unit."

Step-by-step advances are being made in the war against the great killer of newborns, respiratory distress syndrome (RDS).

At the University of Pennsylvania, Dr. Maria Delivoria-Papadopoulas and associates have exchanged the blood of RDS newborns with fresh adult blood. The adult blood has different "oxygen-bonding" characteristics; it releases oxygen to the baby's tissues far easier than does his own blood. "We see a fascinating phenomenon," says Dr. Delivoria-Papadopoulas enthusiastically. "We can *see* the baby's lungs opening up, we can see blood-gases improvement and color improvement. We can see the *baby* improving!" In-utero transfusions to prevent RDS completely are being tested by the team in animal experiments.

In cooperation with physicians at Massachusetts General Hospital, M.I.T. chemical engineer J. Bert Bunnell has devised a means of fighting RDS with artificial surfactant to be inhaled by the infant. Already the lecithin aerosol therapy has saved one RDS baby believed to be near death.

And at Johns Hopkins medical center, an external artificial lung developed by Dr. Theodore Kolobow of the National Heart and Lung Institute kept one 2.2-pound RDS newborn fully supplied with oxygenated blood for seven days. "It was an amazing thing," said one doctor, "before resumption of spontaneous respiration, to see an infant suckling and moving without breathing."

Dr. James suggests that much development is needed in care of babies weighing less than 2.2 pounds. So far, he says, NICUs have had little impact on the survival of infants this small.

For these tiny bits of humanity, artificial wombs are on the way. At the University of Southern California and other institutions, this ultimate NICU is already under development.

Dr. Geoffrey Chamberlain, at King's College Hospital in London, has kept a twenty-six-week-old fetus alive for five hours, as he lay submerged, unbreathing, in a saline water bath. A heart-lung machine oxygenated the blood which was circulated to and from the fetal newborn through a segment of intact umbilical cord.

At the National Heart Institute in Bethesda, Maryland, an artificial womb has sustained some twenty-five fetal lambs for periods ranging up to fifty-five hours.

Proof of success for an artificial womb will come when researchers not only prove they can stave off immediate death. The newborn fetus must actually grow and develop in the new womb in normal fashion.

After witnessing the wave of recent developments in newborn care, can we really say it can't happen— and soon?

CHAPTER

X

Surgery in Miniature

A rare condition threatened Billie shortly after his birth in a Chicago hospital. Something was missing from his body; but until a generation ago no one knew what that something might be, and Billie's life could have ended in weeks—or days.

Billie's large intestine failed to work normally. All of the nerves that normally activate the colon were missing in the final portion of his lower bowel, so that the segment was an inert tube. A blockage developed. The bowel above began to enlarge, gradually causing Billie's abdomen to swell.

At this point Billie's doctor and parents transferred him to the best possible place for him: Chicago's Children's Memorial Hospital. It is one of the world's leading children's hospitals, with full-time staff specialists in children's diseases. Furthermore, its chief of surgery for many years has been Dr. Orvar Swenson, who back in 1947 unraveled the mechanism of Billie's condition, known as Hirschsprung's disease, and developed the operation that is now universally used to cure it.

A correct diagnosis of Hirschsprung's disease is not always easy to make. About 40 percent of the babies who have the condition still die, says Dr. Swenson, because they are misdiagnosed or not diagnosed in time.

Once at Children's Hospital, Billie came under the care of Dr. Joseph O. Sherman, one of the approximately three hundred pediatric surgeons in the United States. A special breed, pediatric surgeons are uniquely qualified to operate on the newborn, to work with tiny instruments and minute infusions, on miniature organs and structures, to correct conditions seldom or never seen by the average general surgeon.

Dr. Sherman ordered a barium enema, which showed that while the diseased portion of the colon was of normal size, the normal portion above it was grossly swollen (because of the blockage). A piece of the lower bowel wall, taken by rectal biopsy and examined under the microscope, showed none of the ganglion cells that form part of the system innervating the normal bowel. This was the final tip-off. Dr. Sherman scheduled an operation for the next morning at 9:30.

"What we'll do," explained Dr. Sherman, "will be in two steps. Tomorrow morning we'll operate through an incision in the abdomen, pull out a loop of large bowel, and do a colostomy. The good bowel will then empty through a hole in the abdomen, into a "cummerbund" diaper. When the child weighs about twenty pounds, at six to eight months of age, we'll do the definitive operation. We'll remove all of the defective lower bowel, below the colostomy, right down to the perineum, the anus. We'll take the good bowel above, pull that through [the operation is known as the Swenson pull-through procedure, after Dr. Orvar Swenson], and attach it below. Assuming that we have no complications from surgery—a very slight chance —this child will lead a normal life, as if he never had the condition."

The next morning, the sleeping seven-pound Billie was wheeled in an incubator into the operating room where Dr. Sherman and his crew awaited, and was placed on a small operating table. Although naked, he lay on a heated mattress and was bathed by heat lamps. Such precautions are essential for a newborn, whose surface area is proportionately larger than an adult's and whose system can be affected drastically by chilling.

On either side of Billie's chest was a silver-dollar-sized electrode to measure his heart function. A tube placed in his throat continuously took his temperature, which was displayed prominently on a large gauge nearby. A metal plate coated with sticky fluid was placed beneath his back to complete the circuit for an electrical instrument that would be used in the operation.

Manning the monitors was the anesthesiologist, who administered small amounts of halothane through a face mask and kept track of Billie's depth of slumber by noting the instinctive clenching of his fist. If the fist is relaxed entirely, the anesthesia is too deep; if the fist is tight, it's not enough.

Billie's abdomen was scrubbed and swabbed. Dr. Sherman helped a nurse place an intravenous catheter into a neck vein. An infusion pump started dripping a glucose-electrolyte fluid into the vein, at a rate of only a few drops per minute.

Finally Billie was draped and the operation began.

Dr. Sherman, using a scalpel with a blade only half an inch long, cut a thin red line two and one-half inches long through the first delicate layer of skin, then through the subcutaneous fat—a leaf of red and white dots. Following behind the knife with an electric cauterizer, second-year resident Edward Smith, M.D., sealed with a sizzle each tiny blood vessel as it was opened by the knife.

Through layer after layer the surgeon cut, finally reaching tough fascia—a sheet of connective tissue—which he severed with a scissors, then the strong muscle layer, into which he made a deep cleft. Beneath the muscle lay more fascia and peritoneum, the tissue lining the abdominal cavity. Once that was cut, a section of Billie's distended large intestine, big as a man's thumb, ballooned out of the opening. Dr. Sherman placed a glass rod under the loop, held it down with his fingers, sliced a bit off so it could be verified by the pathologist as healthy nerve-bearing colon that should be retained, then started to stitch together the opening he had made.

In a few minutes the pathologist returned with his report: the sample was normal; the operation could proceed as planned.

Using black silk threads and curved needles like barbless fishhooks, Dr. Sherman sutured the walls of the ballooned-out, upside-down U of the large intestine to the layers of incised tissue around it. In eight to twelve hours, the end of the loop would be opened to create a *stoma*, a hole, through which fecal matter would drain into the cummerbund diaper. Billie's mother would have two diapers to change instead of just one; otherwise she would handle him like any normal baby. And in the summer, the second stage of the operation would occur, eliminating the stoma.

Finally Dr. Sherman completed the last stitch. The operation had taken one hour. Billie was wrapped warmly and carried, still under the watchful eye of the anesthesiologist, to the intensive-care nursery. One week later he was at home with his mother and father and brothers, and the following summer, on schedule, he was surgically corrected for normal bowel function.

In infant surgery, everything is on a very small scale, especially the subject. A newborn's heart, for example, may be only two inches wide and three inches long. His liver is one-twentieth as big as it will be when he is five, his brain one-third as large.

Pediatric surgeons may use an operating microscope, with a magnification up to forty, to join a minute artery or dissect a tiny structure. Some surgeons wear small binoculars on their eyeglasses.

The operating table is small. Sutures are finer; scissors and forceps are scaled down.

Critical measurements must be made to administer just the right amounts of fluid to such a small patient. A four-and-one-half-pound premature baby contains only five and one-half ounces of blood. During an operation, sponges are weighed to measure blood loss and the baby is periodically given blood transfusions of one-sixth to one-third of an ounce to keep blood volume stable.

The physiology of a baby is unique.

"Medically, one can't look at a baby as a small adult," says Dr. Sherman. "The techniques we use, the problems we run into with an infant are completely different. An example would be sepsis, or overwhelming infection. An adult who gets sepsis has a high temperature and shaking chills. A baby might be lethargic, have a low temperature, and jaundice. Furthermore, the child gets sicker faster (and also gets well quicker, when the corner is turned)."

"If a surgeon is skilled at taking appendices out of adults," says Dr. Robert E. Replogle, chief of pediatric surgery at Wyler Children's Hospital, University of Chicago, "certainly he's OK to do the same for an eight-year-old. When the patient is above a certain size, it doesn't really make a great deal of difference. But it's a whole new ball game when you're talking about these little babies that you can hold in the palm of your hand. Consequently, pediatric surgeons from the beginning of the subspecialty—begun only forty years ago, by Harvard's William E. Ladd and developed by his successor, Robert E. Gross—focused especially on the newborn. In this area, they became very skilled." (Ladd and Gross trained many of today's pediatric surgeons; some ten medical schools at present provide training in pediatric surgery.)

"It's not only the expertise of the pediatric surgeon that counts," adds Dr. Sherman. "Working alone, I couldn't do a good job. You need a good neonatal intensive-care unit like we have here. You need nurses and physicians trained specifically to take care of newborn babies, and pediatric anesthesiologists. It's the whole newborn-care milieu here that makes the difference."

At Children's Memorial Hospital, where half of all cases are surgical, "the trend is subspecialization," explains Dr. Orvar Swenson. "This has been my doing. The urologists here devote all their time to children, as do the orthopedic surgeons, the neurosurgeons, ophthalmologists, and plastic surgeon. You're much better off having a fellow who's doing the same kind of work all the time."

Are all the babies in this country operated on by the right people?

"It's getting better every year," replies Dr. Swenson. "You can't have these high-priced setups all over. But now they're connected with every medical school. And the medical schools are distributed around the country. So it's practical to get babies into medical centers where they can be operated on by pediatric surgeons."

Many surgical problems that occur in newborns are never seen in adults. The reason is simple. They are incompatible with life. The patient is either operated on shortly after birth or never lives to reach adulthood.

Among these unique targets of pediatric surgery are imperforate anus, which prevents defecation; intestinal obstructions; tracheoesophageal fistula, a developmental defect in which usually the upper esophagus ends in a blind pouch while the lower segment opens into the trachea; atresia of the small or large intestine, in which a segment of the intestine is completely missing; and Hirschsprung's disease.

Some anomalies are bizarre, but completely correctible.

When Gary was born, in a small city in Idaho, the delivering physician was aghast to see much of the baby's intestine hanging outside his body. Early in the developmental process Gary's abdominal wall had failed to close, permitting his intestines to slip outside. And now there wasn't room inside for them.

No surgeon in town had had experience with such a condition, known as gastroschisis, which happens only once in every 15,000 births. Until as recently as seven or eight years ago, 90 percent of its victims died; today, with pediatric surgery, 80 percent can be saved. As Gary's condition worsened, a telephone call from his pediatrician resulted in a flying rescue by the Intermountain Newborn Intensive Care Center at the

University of Utah Medical Center. Once at the center, Gary was operated on by a pediatric surgeon who put all of the extra bowel into a Dacron sack and attached it to the abdominal cavity. Each day he stuffed a bit more of the intestine inside, gradually stretching the perineal cavity until the intestine was completely inside and functioning perfectly. Then he sewed up Gary, who today is normal in every respect.

Heart defects are among the most frequently occurring life-threatening birth anomalies. Long thought to be random accidents, they are now known to fall into a relatively few specific patterns—a fact elucidated during the 1940s in the writings of Johns Hopkins' Dr. Helen Taussig, best known as the co-originator of the first successful blue-baby operation.

Specific operations have been developed to deal with the great majority of heart malformations. Thus, the blue-baby operation (so-called because the baby was blue from lack of oxygen) involved creation of an artificial shunt to increase the flow of blood from the heart to the lungs.

Most common of the 30,000 infant heart defects requiring surgery each year is patent ductus arteriosus. The condition affects only one term baby in 250, and but one premature in seven. If severe enough, it produces symptoms that require surgery: cessation of breathing, increasing concentration of carbon dioxide in the blood, or accentuation of respiratory distress.

Before birth, the short blood vessel known as the patent ductus performs a useful function. It connects the aorta and the pulmonary artery, the two major blood vessels leading out of the heart; it shunts blood from the aorta to the pulmonary artery, permitting most of the fetal circulation to bypass the lungs. Normally, the ductus closes completely ten to fifteen hours after birth; as the level of oxygen in the new-born's blood rises, the inner lining of the patent ductus contracts, gradually pinching the vessel shut. If the ductus fails to close after a few hours or days, perhaps because of the immaturity of the newborn or insufficient oxygen in the blood, the baby is in real trouble.

Johnnie weighed just a bit more than two pounds when he was born at the Los Angeles County–University of Southern California Medical Center. Despite his weight and his gestational age of only thirty to thirty-one weeks, he looked healthy and seemed free of problems until his eighth day of life. Then he stopped breathing, and was resuscitated, something that was to happen again—and again. A mechanical respirator brought to his side began to breathe for him.

Examining him in the newborn intensive-care unit, neonatologist Dr. Joan Hodgman detected a large murmur characteristic of patent ductus arteriosus. Much of Johnnie's blood simply was detouring around his lungs. Furthermore, the shunting created an overload of blood for the heart; Johnnie was in the throes of gross congestive heart failure.

Digitalis and diuretics were given during the next forty-eight to seventy-two hours, but the heart failure did not improve. Studies in the meantime confirmed that a large part of Johnnie's blood was shunting left to right through his patent ductus.

The odds against Johnnie seemed tremendous—the risk of being so premature and small, of congestive heart failure, of insufficient oxygen in the blood. An operation would be necessary, posing still an additional risk for the patient who now, having deteriorated, weighed only 1.8 pounds.

All of this was explained to Johnnie's parents, who

agreed to the operation, by Dr. Arnold Coran, chief of pediatric surgery at the medical center.

With Dr. Coran, at this medical center, Johnnie had the best possible chance to pull through. Dr. Coran, thirty-four, trained at Boston Children's Hospital under the originator of the patent ductus operation, Dr. Robert E. Gross. Doctors at Los Angeles County, because of the huge volume of births at the center, says Coran, "probably have more experience, operating on tiny babies, than surgeons at any other place in the world. We operate on one hundred newborns a year, of which seventy-five are prematures. Last year we performed thirty patent ductus operations—more than one every other week."

The next morning, when Johnnie was eleven days old, the operation began. Dr. Coran cut into Johnnie's chest on the left side, then employed small retractors to spread two ribs apart. Through the opening went the scalpel of Dr. Coran, who soon had exposed Johnnie's enlarged patent ductus. "In these tiny babies it's very large, larger than the aorta itself," noted Dr. Coran to student observers. Dimly visible through the walls of the whitish vessel was the bright red oxygenated blood pulsing through it, being shunted uselessly around in a lung-to-heart-to-lung circle rather than coursing out to the body tissues in need of it. Dr. Coran dissected the patent ductus free of surrounding tissue, then tied two large black silk ligatures around it, on either end, pulling the thread tightly to seal off the vessel. The essential part of the operation was thus performed. Soon Dr. Coran and his assisting resident surgeon had closed the chest and the operation was finished. It had taken twenty-seven minutes.

Almost immediately Johnnie's skin became pinker; he began to improve, for the operation had given him instantly a normal circulation pattern. Twelve hours after surgery, the respirator mask was taken off Johnnie's face and he began to breathe on his own, without added oxygen. Less and less digitalis was given to him; in a few days it was stopped altogether. Johnnie remained in the hospital nursery, just in case anything went wrong (which it didn't) until he weighed five pounds. Ten weeks after the operation, he went home to his delighted parents.

Surgery on the inner parts of a baby's heart could not be performed until the 1950s. There was no way to stop the heart, do an operation, and keep the patient alive. Then, in 1953, Dr. C. Walton Lillehei at the University of Minnesota effectively bypassed the heart by using the baby's mother or father as a living heart-lung machine. The mother or father, whichever had blood that matched the baby's, lay on a table beside the infant; the parent's blood was pumped to the baby and the baby's blood back to the parent, whose lungs oxygenated it.

Then came the heart-lung machine itself, which worked very well for adult open-heart surgery. A pediatric version, one-sixth the adult size, was effective for small children, but nothing particularly suited the newborn, especially the premature. The tubes leading to and from the heart, little bigger than the baby's fist, got in the way of the operation; and circulation of the blood through the machine seemed to damage the corpuscles.

In the early 1960s Dr. Y. Hikasa and associates at Japan's Kyoto University operated successfully on scores of tiny infants by cooling their bodies down to 60 degrees Fahrenheit, in effect placing them in a kind of suspended animation. Using the heart-lung machine only minimally, the Japanese surgeons achieved a still, relaxed, bloodless heart on which they could operate for at least one half hour (without apparent brain damage to the infant). Surgeons around the world picked up the technique, devising their own individual modifications. With it, among other things, they could repair heart valves, stitch up holes within the heart, and correct transposition of the great vessels of the heart. No longer was it always necessary to wait for a baby to grow big enough to be operated on, a wait that frequently was fatal.

In the operating room of the University of Chicago's chief pediatric surgeon, Dr. Robert Replogle, a three-week-old infant lies packed in plastic bags of ice, cooling down for the operation. The baby is anesthetized with ether.

After an hour of cooling, by which time the baby's temperature has dropped to 64 degrees, its heart from 180 to 25 beats per minute, Dr. Replogle begins to cut into the chest wall. Once Replogle exposes the heart and prepares for subsequent connection to the heart-lung machine, a paralyzing solution is injected into the tiny, rapidly pulsating organ. The beat dies away; the heart lies still. Dr. Replogle opens the heart, carves out a two-ounce tumor that had almost completely filled a chamber, then repairs the incisions he has made. As soon as he stitches up the heart itself, he jolts the heart electrically, restarting its previous regular motion. Connections are made to a heart-lung machine to assist the heart and rewarm the patient. The baby resumes breathing.

In three years, using this method, Dr. Replogle has operated on some three dozen infants, including another with a tumor of the heart. Despite its risks and limitations, he believes it presents the most opportunity to make certain operations safer to perform.

Not always is the scalpel the operating tool, nor will it be in the future. It may at times be a laser beam, a freezing tool, or even a hypodermic needle.

Using a metal syringe, Dr. Robert A. Good in 1968 saved the life of seven-month-old David Camp of Meriden, Connecticut. David was born with a rare, inherited blood disease of which there were no known survivors. He had no immunity system, no antibodies to fight off bacteria or viruses.

Immunologist Good, then of the University of Minnesota, employed a hollow needle to withdraw two ounces of bone marrow from a hip bone of David Camp's nine-year-old sister, and, with a different needle, injected the marrow into David's abdominal cavity. The marrow cells, which in a normal person manufacture antibodies, were picked up by David's bloodstream, which carried them to the marrow of David's bones. A later injection completely changed David's blood type to that of his sister. Within David's bones antibody-producing marrow cells began to grow, and his condition was cured.

Other doctors have repeated Dr. Good's success. In the future, as many as twenty presently fatal inherited blood diseases may be treated with the technique.

What has been the greatest recent advance in pediatric surgery? I asked Dr. Orvar Swenson.

"Undoubtedly," he said, "it has been the ability to feed a baby completely intravenously."

To keep a baby alive and operate on him when he's bigger, rather than right away?

"Well, yes, it could be used that way, but it really is most valuable when a baby is really sick and has a combination of things that prevents the intestine from working. This could be severe—peritonitis, infection, or it could be a mechanical obstruction. It's used mostly when you get into a jam postoperatively.

"For a long time, we could give babies and adults water and salt (electrolytes) intravenously, but we couldn't give them enough calories to maintain normal growth and development. There's no fat you can give intravenously, and if you tried to give enough calories with a dilute sugar solution alone, you would flood the baby with fluid.

"Everybody said, you can't give a sugar concentration stronger than five or ten percent—and it's true, if you give it in a vein, in the arm, the stronger solution causes the vein to clog shut within twenty-four hours.

"Then a surgeon at the University of Pennsylvania, Stanley Dudrick, was young enough not to believe what everybody said, that you can't give a hypertonic solution [more than 10 percent sugar]. He put a catheter in a vein of a dog and threaded it down until it was next to the heart, to the vena cava where the volume of blood is large. And he put a very concentrated solution in there and got by with it.

"This solution contained twenty-five-percent glucose. Then he added protein hydrolysate which gave protein, and he had a solution which supplied the total caloric needs.

"Dudrick tried it on baby animals and then infants and kept them alive and growing—something never before possible. And now this new method is employed worldwide."

Like some other advances in medicine, parenteral hyperalimentation, as it is called, by its success has created a tragic dilemma.

"I call it the therapeutic toboggan," says Dr. Swenson. "We're so well endowed today with antibiotics, surgical techniques, artificial respiration, and feeding that we can keep even a hopeless patient alive. You start, and you never know when to quit.

"We've got a baby upstairs who illustrates this." (I had just seen her—small for her age of eight months, looking a bit sad but bright-eyed, going back and forth in a motor-driven toddler's swing to which was attached the intravenous bottle that continually nourished her.)

"This baby came into the neurosurgical service because of mild hydrocephalus, and then became septic, infected. The neurosurgeon said, 'We don't dare put a shunt in (to drain off the excess fluid on the brain), because of the septic condition.'

"Then it developed that the child had a perforated intestine, an acute problem. So we went in to correct that and found the colon in very bad condition. Right then arose the question: are you going to give up? Well, the fellows decided, no, we'll give the baby fluids orally, and lo and behold, she survived. Then it got to the point where you couldn't feed the baby orally. So they tried predigested feedings and that didn't work. Then they went to hyperalimentation.

"So now, for months, we've kept the baby alive with hyperalimentation. The hydrocephalus has stabilized so an operation won't be necessary. We'll get the intestine fixed up—I think. She has fifty-percent viable colon, which will probably be enough to reconstruct her. She's starting to take oral feedings again. We'll probably make it with this child—but we were very, very close to facing the problem that arose with one of the very first babies kept alive by hyperalimentation: almost all of that baby's small intestine had been destroyed by disease. Hyperalimentation kept him living for eighteen months, but then, you know, they had to do something. They tried feeding the baby and he didn't have enough intestine and they had to let him die."

He could have been kept alive for years?

"Probably. But what would you have done? I think one of our real problems today is to know when you're licked. I personally feel that if you've got too bad a situation you should not do extraordinary things, such as using a respirator to breathe for them, and using hyperalimentation."

A somewhat different view comes from Dr. Robert Replogle.

"The public tells us," says Replogle, "that the doctor should establish when the situation is hopeless, and at that time withhold further heroic treatment.

"There is a distinct and important difference between withholding treatment in a 'hopeless' case and doing something active that may lead to death. In the former situation, 'hopeless' may be difficult to define, and the physician finds himself grasping for any kind of straw that may help him justify keeping the patient alive. Our mission primarily is to save life, and it is very difficult to go against your own professional and personal instincts. Most doctors agree that a patient should have the right to a dignified death, and making heroic efforts at saving life in a 'hopeless' situation seems to be of little virtue. On the other hand, actively promoting death is an entirely different proposition. This is a question that the public needs to answer. The doctor has a contract with the patient to get him well. It's a hundred-percent contract, in my mind, without any fine print.

"Now, the public may want to define what our priorities are. What is it we're trying to do? Are we trying to make everybody live to be a thousand? To make everybody live to be eighty and be happy? Is it to save every little baby with every horrible kind of deformity? Can we spend a thousand dollars of public money to save an infant's life? One hundred thousand?"

"I want to make it clear," adds Dr. Swenson, "that as long as a baby has the potential for a fairly normal existence, I believe there should be no limits on what we do to save life. What troubles us is the patient with a badly damaged brain or one who has no chance of functioning adequately because of neuromuscular defects."

What will be the next great development in the future of newborn surgery?

"Transplants," says Dr. Swenson, "once we find a better way of controlling the problem of the body rejecting the transplanted organ. Rejection is still a great problem even with kidney transplants, which have been more successful than others. The patient must stay on immunity-suppressing drugs as long as he lives, or the immune mechanisms come roaring back and kick that kidney right out. Meanwhile, the patient is susceptible to any disease that comes along.

"Heart transplants would be the greatest need in newborns. There are quite a few uncorrectable heart conditions—and partial corrections that just drag on. If you could give them a new heart, you'd be far ahead of the game."

Dr. Robert Replogle believes "We'll go from the stage of newborn surgery such as we have now—plus perhaps some fetal surgery, including heart repair—to the stage of not having the problems of congenital disease. We'll figure out ways to avoid them, but that is a long way away, certainly not in the next decade. Surgery, you know, although the best solution to many current physical problems, isn't really the ultimate answer to anything."

The process of avoiding congenital birth defects has already started, says Children's Memorial's Dr. Sherman.

"Many of the birth defects we repair surgically are not inherited," he points out. "They are *caused*—some perhaps by certain drugs, some because of reasons that have to do with the age of the mother. For example, a mother past thirty-five has a greater chance of bearing a damaged child, as do girls of thirteen, fourteen, and fifteen. Why we don't really know.

"But the Pill has affected our practice here. Births under unfavorable circumstances are avoided. In the future, effective birth control and the use of amniocentesis with subsequent therapeutic abortions will decrease the number of birth defects."

Dr. Sherman and his counterparts in medical centers across the nation do not expect to run out of work soon. For tomorrow and the next day and the next will surely come another call to save a tiny life at its very beginning.

CHAPTER

XI

Getting the Best Care

Having a physician attend a pregnancy and birth is like fire insurance. Most of the time it doesn't matter what kind of fire insurance you have or even if you have it. It doesn't matter, that is, unless you have a fire. Then you need insurance in the worst way and you want and need the very best kind.

Similarly, as happened for thousands of years, the vast majority of births would turn out perfectly well without a physician or a hospital. The only justification for either is as insurance against the unusual or the unexpected.

How does a mother-to-be obtain the best "birth insurance," the best possible doctor, the best hospital? While interviewing experts for this book, I kept trying to find out. And some of the answers were surprising.

The first question seemed easy. Which is better, a GP or an obstetrician? But even this simple query did not have an obvious, clear-cut answer.

A physician's *interest in obstetrics* is as important as

anything else, according to obstetrician Jack M. Schneider, M.D., codirector of the University of Wisconsin's perinatal center. And because a doctor is a specialist in obstetrics-gynecology doesn't mean he really likes to outline diets and deliver babies. His special training is often surgery, with gynecology as his chief interest.

"Some GPs I know do a better job than some obstetricians. Statistically, it is safer in our region to be delivered by a GP in a small hospital, if that hospital has ties with a regional perinatal center, than to be managed by a specialist in an independent nonperinatal center hospital.

"The main things that cause infant mortality are as well known to the knowledgeable GP as they are to the specialist. And they're as poorly known and understood by the lackluster specialist or GP. If an obstetrician-gynecologist cares for obstetrical cases because he *has* to—and there are some who don't like to get up at night, who would rather do surgery—they tend not to keep up with obstetrical advances. It's the same story with a GP who runs his legs off doing pediatrics, but dislikes obstetrics."

Another obstetrician advises, "Most of all it depends upon finding someone who knows his limits, accepts them, acts upon them. I don't care what degree he has on the wall."

How do you find a doctor interested in obstetrics?

Ask neighbors and friends for recommendations; ask them to tell you about their experiences. Ask your prospective doctor how many babies he delivers a year; two hundred is a good load for a specialist, while three hundred may be almost too many, depending upon other commitments.

"You can't make rigid rules that say 'All patients

with this go there," says Dr. Michael Hartigan, a pediatrician-neonatologist of La Crosse, Wisconsin. "I would say that if a mother-to-be has a complication that puts her into the high-risk category, at least a consultation should be sought from those people most expert in a given area. If the patient is a diabetic, for example, or has a heart problem, she should be in the hands of the best-trained man in that field, whether he's a particularly nice guy or not."

Neonatologist John Grausz, M.D., Milwaukee, suggests that a woman ask her doctor to get a consultation by saying, "I'd like a second opinion on this." The consultation, says Grausz, should come from the nearest medical school medical center, not from the man's partner or friend. "Obstetricians," says Grausz, "don't usually consult with each other. They are much more likely just to go ahead and let time solve the problem. And that's where the high-risk case goes off the rails."

This request for consultation, says Grausz, "might make your doctor very mad. If this happens, you don't want him anyway; doctors have no business getting angry at patients seeking good care."

Dr. Hartigan recommends a frank discussion between patient and doctor before she becomes pregnant. "The approach should be—let's sit down and have an agreement. Let's clear up all possible questions at the beginning. Because if someone quizzes me all through the care, then I think she needs another doctor. Because she obviously doesn't trust me. And trust is a lot of what we're talking about."

Ideally, selection of a physician to deliver one's babies should come long before pregnancy—perhaps when a woman is married and moves to a new community. It might not be convenient to look for a new doctor at the onset of pregnancy. A health problem might require treatment *before* pregnancy; the doctor should be advised ahead of time of pregnancy plans.

The affiliations of a doctor are important in judging his competence. To find out if an obstetrician is board-certified, write to the American College of Obstetricians and Gynecologists, 1 Wacker Drive, Chicago, Ill. Write to the American Academy of Family Physicians, Volker Blvd. at Brookside Blvd., Kansas City, Mo. 64112, to discover if a GP (or "family practitioner") has maintained his continuing education with postgraduate study. He must, to retain his board certification in family practice.

The hospital in which a doctor practices is crucial in determining what kind of care he can provide you. Choose a doctor who admits his patients to a hospital accredited by the Joint Committee on Accreditation of Hospitals, 645 N. Michigan Ave., Chicago, Ill. 60611. One-third of all American hospitals are not so accredited. If possible, choose a teaching hospital, one with a medical school affiliation. It is more likely to have a skilled nursing staff and twenty-four-hour coverage by resident M.D.s who can deliver your baby even if your doctor doesn't make it or is delayed. Choose a hospital that permits any procedures you might desire, a point that will be expanded upon later.

It is best if your doctor is in group practice, with at least two other obstetrically qualified physicians to cover for him at night and on weekends. Sometimes each doctor takes a twenty-four-hour shift, sleeping at the hospital between deliveries. Thus, while your baby may not be delivered by the doctor of your choice, whatever doctor attends you in the office and at the hospital won't be hung over from lack of sleep.

If you are new in town, and have a family doctor,

ask him for recommendations. Or if you are moving to a new town, ask your present doctor to give you a name.

You *could* call up the local county medical society and ask for a recommendation, but they will not recommend one of their members over another. They will just give you the names of two or three members who deliver babies, a selection taken from the top of a rotating list.

While choosing a doctor to handle a pregnancy, it's wise to seek recommendations regarding a pediatrician for the newborn. Stanley Harrison, M.D., of the American Academy of Pediatrics suggests that you ask your family doctor; ask mothers you know; find a doctor who is on the staff of the nearest children's hospital; telephone the local chapter of the American Academy of Pediatrics and get a few names of members, all of whom will be board-certified. Write the academy at 1801 Hinman Ave., Evanston, Ill. 60201. Or call the county medical society and ask them to give you some names of board-certified pediatricians.

One good way to choose a competent doctor is to telephone the dean of the nearest medical school and ask for a recommendation.

Is the doctor right for *you?* Does he take time to answer questions to your satisfaction? If you want to use the Lamaze method of prepared childbirth, will he go along with it or "knock you out" at the last minute? If you want to breast-feed, will he encourage and support you, or scoff at you? Talk to him, and ask his patients.

Is the doctor "new wave" or "status quo"? Is he abreast of or at least aware of the recent revolutionary obstetric advances discussed in this book? (Don't expect him to know *everything*; his attitude is what's most important.) Does he hold a position on the staff of the nearest medical school? (If so, he is more likely to keep up with new developments.)

Complications may necessitate a reevaluation of your medical care. Certain procedures are best done by specialists at a medical center. Thus, points out Dr. Karlis Adamsons, of New York's Mount Sinai Hospital, doctors in private practice just don't have enough volume to get good at certain things. "A doctor who delivers two hundred babies a year has only about five-percent complicated cases, or ten per year. That's not much of an experience. Whereas, if a doctor is in charge of the complicated pregnancy clinic of a university hospital, or any hospital delivering two thousand to ten thousand patients, he develops a totally different degree of expertise.

"This was well documented when the first fetal transfusions were started. The results were discouragingly poor. And then as groups gained more experience, it became obvious that it was not the transfusion that was intrinsically dangerous or difficult, it was just the burdens of the inexperienced hand. After a while those who continued in this field of medical therapy developed skills and confidence in the procedure that no longer made it hazardous, either to mother or fetus."

Within the next several years, predicts Dr. Edward J. Quilligan of the University of Southern California, every major obstetric unit will include on its staff a new kind of expert to act as a consultant to obstetricians. (Dr. Quilligan serves on a board setting up standards for certifying this superspecialist.) He will be a "specialist in maternal and fetal medicine" whose attention is concentrated in just that field. Today, only a few medical centers have someone so qualified. "In practice, at present, the obstetrician handling a complicated case calls in an internist or occasionally a pediatrician and together they jointly manage the patient."

A medical school may have on its staff a person who specializes in a certain kind of pregnancy problem. Thus, Dr. John Grausz tells of a woman he knows who had lost nine pregnancies in a row, who had no living children, but ended up as the patient of a miscarriage specialist at the Medical College of Wisconsin. "She spent much time in bed, had all kinds of medications, and carried the baby to term. With the next two pregnancies and the same doctor, she followed the same procedures and now has three healthy children."

The choice of a hospital frequently depends upon what doctor one has chosen, and which hospital he delivers in. Thus it probably is wisest to choose the hospital first, and the doctor second.

How big should a hospital be?

There are different opinions. A veteran obstetrical nurse says, "The small hospitals (in small towns) do a better job for the average uncomplicated case. The mother knows the nurses. The doctor knows the father. The father can come and go."

But Dr. Ben Peckham, chief of gynecology-obstetrics at the University of Wisconsin, says that "The real difficulty with the small hospitals is that they're not really set up to take care of even the average patient. The average patient who was perfectly uncomplicated before she went into labor can get complicated awfully fast."

What is small? "Any with total deliveries of less than five hundred a year. Particularly when it's staffed by people who are not specializing in obstetrics, this is just a part-time, oftentimes not a very desirable aspect of practice that's required of them because there's nobody else around to do it. So the nurse gets stuck with watching these patients and really doing everything including delivering them at times because the doctor's too busy to get there. So she's left quite untrained or not even necessarily experienced to deal with a problem that can become very technically demanding."

Dr. Sprague Gardiner, recent president of the American College of Obstetricians and Gynecologists (ACOG), says, "I think it's been pretty well shown that unless a hospital has a thousand deliveries or more per year it can't really afford to support the personnel and equipment needed to provide really quality care."

A 1967 national study by ACOG found that the most deficiencies in maternity care were associated with small hospital size, few deliveries per year, and lack of teaching affiliations. Some examples of deficiencies found by the study: 25 percent of hospitals required more than forty minutes to prepare for an emergency Cesarean section; 43 percent couldn't administer blood within less than thirty minutes' notice; and 30 percent required more than four hours to prepare for an exchange transfusion. Other defects: absence of a separate recovery room after delivery; lack of continuous observation (of mother and infant) in the first hour following delivery; limited availability of anesthesiologists, nurse-anesthetists and X ray technicians; infrequent administration of hemoglobin and urine tests before delivery; and failure to make a complete examination of the newborn.

Dr. Gardiner predicts that eventually there will be

three or four different types of hospitals. "The largest center would have the whole works. It would be a complete perinatal center. There would be a high-risk maternity clinic, newborn intensive-care nursery, round-the-clock laboratory and blood bank, genetic counseling, all the advanced equipment for monitoring and the like. This unit might deliver five thousand babies a year.

"Then you'd have another level of hospital with staff and equipment to provide quality care. There would be intensive-care units. But there wouldn't be as many facilities or consultative resources. This hospital might have two thousand deliveries annually.

"A third type of hospital, for remote, rural regions only, would have a minimal number of parameters to measure patients in labor and the immediate newborn. If the patients run into trouble, they could be transported if necessary—either the mother or baby—to a center that has more facilities. Minimum deliveries would be five hundred babies a year."

Consideration should be given to hospital rules that may affect the handling of your case. In general, Catholic hospitals tend to be most restrictive in banning certain procedures. Catholic hospitals account for 29 percent of the hospital beds in this country; one-third of them serve U.S. communities with no other health services. But their rules apply to Catholics and non-Catholics alike within their walls. At this writing, all U.S. Catholic hospitals prohibit abortion, sterilization as a means of contraception, artificial insemination, and curettage of the endometrium (scraping of the inner lining of the uterus) after rape to prevent embryo implantation.

Thus, a woman who desires a tubal ligation right after delivery, a time when the tubes are readily acces-

sible and the operation is easy, when she can save the
time and expense of a separate hospitalization, should
not deliver at a Catholic hospital. Similarly, some unnecessary hysterectomies take place at Catholic hospitals as an indirect means of sterilization. Indirect sterilization procedures are permitted when they are
"immediately directed to the cure, diminution or prevention of a serious pathological condition and are not
directly contraceptive" in the words of the "Ethical
and Religious Directives for Catholic Health Facilities" approved by the National Conference of Catholic Bishops of the United States.

The directives, predicts Anthony R. Kosnik, dean of
theology at Ss. Cyril and Methodius Seminary, are
going to force Catholic hospitals to abandon some
areas of service. Some Catholic hospitals under construction, he says, have eliminated maternity units as
a result of the proclamation.

Other hospital rules have nothing to do with reli-
gion or ethics, but affect the support the husband is
allowed to give his wife during the birth of their child.
Some hospitals still forbid fathers or other visitors in
the labor rooms; many more shut the father out of the
delivery room.

In the case of premature birth, all other considerations should go out the window, says John Grausz,
M.D., of Milwaukee County Hospital. "If you go into
labor six weeks or more before due date," he advises,
"don't bother with an inadequate facility. For the sake
of the baby and often the mother, forget the community hospital in which you were going to deliver. Call
the emergency squad or police and get yourself rushed
to the nearest perinatal center, if it's reachable. In
metropolitan Milwaukee, for example, with sirens go-

ing, and not allowing for peak-hour traffic, there's no place that's more than fifteen to twenty minutes from this place."

Grausz points out that most Americans today live in large metropolitan areas, or are within an hour's drive of a medical center affiliated with a medical school.

In choosing a doctor or a hospital, it's important to know whether your case would be considered high risk. But what is high risk?

"In the past," says Dr. Grausz, "high risk was a static thing—a diagnosis, like diabetes. There was nothing to be done. You made the diagnosis and then sat back and waited for things to happen.

"To me high risk is a red flag. It's a call to action. It's a call to changing gears on this particular patient. It's something that alerts people that here is a case that requires watching, planning, foresight, managing, and an understanding of what bad things might happen. When anything goes wrong, the doctor has to step in and interrupt the process so the situation goes back on an even keel. You try to change the high risk into a low risk."

Nine out of ten middle-class mothers-to-be are not high risk. Fewer than 10 percent of private patients in the United States fall into this category. But for those who wish to check themselves against a basic high-risk yardstick, a guide follows. The guide and the section, "Where Should You Deliver?" were prepared by the author for *Ladies' Home Journal* (1974) with the assistance of Jack M. Schneider, M.D., who is codirector, Wisconsin Perinatal Center, Madison, Wisconsin, and associate professor, Department of Gynecology-Obstetrics and Pediatrics, University of Wisconsin Center for Health Sciences.

Are You High Risk?

If you are pregnant and fall into any of the categories below, your case is considered high risk by most obstetricians. Special care is needed to diminish or eliminate extra risk to the health of you and/or your baby. Ask your obstetrician to explain what special measures he is taking.

Age of mother
>   Under 16/over 40.

Birth number
>   Sixth or later child.
>   First child to woman thirty-five or older.
>   Twins, triplets, etc. (multiple pregnancy).

History
>   Previous miscarriage or stillbirth.
>   Previous Cesarean delivery.
>   Previous toxemia of pregnancy.
>   Previous premature birth.
>   Previous child weighing over nine pounds (may indicate mother is diabetic) or under five and one-half pounds at birth.
>   Bleeding during previous pregnancies.

Rh factor
>   Rh incompatibility when wife is Rh negative and husband is Rh positive. (Now possible to prevent, to a great extent, by immunizing woman with Rho-gam within hours after each birth or miscarriage.) If mother is already sensitized, amniocentesis and intrauterine blood transfusion may be necessary.

Ill Health of Mother
>   Anemia.

Heart, circulatory, or kidney disease; high blood pressure.

Diabetes. (Requires diet and blood sugar control, possibly early delivery, and strict control of mother's blood sugar in labor. A sample of amniotic fluid is taken to determine when baby is mature enough to deliver.)

Malnutrition (should be corrected *before* pregnancy) or obesity.

Urinary tract infection. (May be cured by medication. Often without symptoms.)

Rubella infection of mother during pregnancy (30 percent to 50 percent of fetuses damaged if this occurs in first three months of pregnancy; therapeutic abortion may be indicated. Can be prevented by vaccination of mother-to-be two months or more *before* she becomes pregnant.)

Emotional instability.

Tuberculosis. (Should be cured by medication before pregnancy.)

Syphilis or gonorrhea. (Can be cured by medication during pregnancy.)

Toxoplasmosis. (An infection carried by animals, especially cats. Most often contracted, however, by eating rare meat.)

Anatomical defects

Android (manlike) pelvis.

Incompetent cervix. (Corrected during pregnancy by minor surgery.)

Genetic problems

Previous offspring, siblings, or ancestors with genetic defect such as Down's syn-

drome or Tay-Sachs disease. (Requires amniocentesis, chromosome analysis.)

Others likely to be at high risk during pregnancy
include drug addicts, heavy smokers or drink-
ers, the unwed or separated or divorced, the
poverty-stricken, anyone under unusual stress.

WHERE SHOULD YOU DELIVER?

High-risk mothers should deliver their babies in a
fully equipped and staffed perinatal center. They
should do this not so much for their own sakes, but for
the sake of the unborn.

Most perinatal centers are the maternity wings and
attached nurseries of large hospitals affiliated with
medical schools. In effect they provide intensive care
for women in labor and for the high-risk babies that
high-risk mothers frequently produce. Fortunately,
especially with proper prenatal care, most high-risk
mothers give birth to healthy babies. And the babies
of some apparently healthy mothers end up premature
or in need of special care. (See, for example, Chapters
IX and XII.)

COMPONENTS OF A PERINATAL CENTER*

I. *Services*
    a. Maternal-fetal intensive-care prenatal
       clinics
    b. Intrapartum maternal-fetal intensive care
    c. Neonatal intensive care

*Prepared by Jack M. Schneider, M.D., Codirector, Wisconsin
Perinatal Center, Madison.

---

    d. Laboratory capabilities to include:
       1. blood-gas studies within 10 minutes
       2. blood bank with blood and fibrinogen available
       3. hematology
       4. 24-hour quality radiology services
    e. Supportive services—anesthesia, respiratory care, resuscitation, genetics, social services
    f. Follow-up clinics—maternal and neonatal

2. *Personnel*
    a. Perinatologists—obstetricians
    b. Neonatologists
    c. Anesthesiologists
    d. Nurse specialists—clinicians trained in maternal-fetal or neonatal intensive care
    e. Others from supportive services

3. *Support Equipment—adequate in number and modern to provide required services*

4. *Quality of care assessment*
    a. Collection/review of data
    b. Peer review of *all* components of care team in center *and* in other hospitals of region served

5. *Education Programs*
    a. Regional (center is responsible for perinatal education in other hospitals it serves)
    b. In-service

One of the features of a complete perinatal center is a "high risk" clinic that manages prenatal care in complicated cases, or assists private physicians in doing so.

Special tests and diagnostic equipment are available, as are all the other resources of a large modern hospital. Medical and nurse consultants, social workers, dieticians, and perhaps even genetic counselors may be called in to help solve a difficult case.

In the modern perinatal center, a staff obstetrician is on duty at all times; laboratory and blood bank facilities can be mobilized at any hour. Obstetric nurses have advanced training in their specialty; some may even have extensive training as modern midwives. Electronic monitors track the heartbeat of the unborn baby and the mother's uterine contractions.

A staff pediatrician joins the delivery team during any birth in which complications are likely to occur, so he can resuscitate the baby if necessary. In the newborn intensive care unit, prematures and critically ill babies are minutely watched—sometimes on a one-to-one basis—by specially trained nurses under the direction of a neonatologist (a subspecialty of pediatrics). The newborns are encased in incubators and attached to electronic monitors, intravenous lines, and sometimes even to machines that breath for them.

Costs

Unfortunately, most parents-to-be in the United States are poorly prepared to meet the costs of high-risk care should it become necessary. Most health insurance does not begin to provide coverage necessary for modern intensive care; it probably will not until forced to change by popular demand or legislation.

Many health insurance policies have a ceiling for maternal care that is even below the cost of *routine* care. Yet, a diabetic mother-to-be may need to be hospitalized for two to eight weeks before delivery, and with laboratory charges the bill may be $200 a *day*.

It is common for health insurance policies to exclude the first fifteen days or even the first thirty days of newborn care; yet this is the period when costs are highest. A bill of $1500 or $2000 for a stay in a newborn intensive-care unit is typical. Costs for a baby while he is on a respirator can run $1000 a week or as high as $500 a day.

Senator Edward M. Kennedy tells about young James Rieger, of Cleveland, and his testimony before Kennedy's Senate Health Subcommittee. While giving birth, Mrs. Rieger suffered a cardiac arrest. She and the baby were in intensive care for two months in Cleveland Metropolitan Hospital, and the bill came to $20,000. All Rieger's insurance paid was $350. Rieger was out of work because of a strike; he was forced into bankruptcy and his automobile, TV, refrigerator, and even the kitchen stove were taken away.

None of these figures obviously should be used as an argument against modern care for mothers and babies; they are small compared with the agonies they prevent, and with the up to $500,000 cost of maintaining a mentally retarded individual (maimed by inadequate care) in an institution for life. But better means must be found to meet costs.

Governmental support of some kind may be forthcoming. In Arizona, for example, the state now pays for the cost of care in a newborn intensive-care unit, in excess of $1000. A recent bill in the California legislature sought to qualify RDS-afflicted babies for state aid-to-crippled-children funds. National health insurance of some kind is on the way, a fact acknowledged even by the medical establishment. But no one at this writing knows what or who it would include.

If you are poor and live in an area served by a really good county hospital, good perinatal care, if available, is "free." (It may also be impersonal and unsupportive, require long waits for prenatal checkups, and exclude the husband.) Thus, in Milwaukee, the poor patient at County Hospital gets the most advanced care in town. According to Joan E. Hodgman, M.D., in 1973, the only true perinatal centers in Los Angeles were at Los Angeles County–University of Southern California Medical Center; Martin Luther King Hospital; and Harbor General Hospital—all county hospitals—and at Cedars of Lebanon, a private hospital. The Kaiser system also provided comprehensive perinatal care.

For parents-to-be reading this book, at this time, better health insurance is the answer to the cost problem. This may require a separate "comprehensive major medical" policy bought through an employer or from an agent. If bought through an employer, it should be one that can be converted to an individual policy and continued after termination of employment.

The insurance should cover catastrophic health expenses—with a maximum of $20,000 or more. It should cover all complications of pregnancy, including care of the unborn child and also care of the newborn baby from birth. There should be no exclusions for laboratory, X ray, anesthesiology, equipment, drug, ambulance, or consultation fees. A deductible figure of at least $500 is necessary, otherwise the policy will cost too much.

Insurance may also be through membership in a health maintenance organization such as a Kaiser-Permanente Plan. These comprehensive prepaid health plans are being established all over the country by Blue Cross, doctors' groups, and major insurance companies, with the support and encouragement of the Federal Government. Coverages of these plans differ, so each policy must be studied individually in terms of perinatal care provided, catastrophic expenses, exclusions, and limits.

CHAPTER

XII

Getting It All Together: Regional Perinatal Care

The time is 1977. On the Lac du Flambeau Indian Reservation deep in Wisconsin's North Woods, pretty Jennie Eagle, eighteen, has recently conceived.

So has Mona Henney, thirty-nine, of suburban Fox Point on Milwaukee's wealthy North Shore. And Jean Tabor, twenty-six, a professor's wife in Madison, Wisconsin, the state capital and seat of its university.

Because of a concept pioneered in Wisconsin and elsewhere as early as 1974, the three pregnancies are equally safeguarded. Each is registered by the attending physician with a regional perinatal center, a kind of superhospital unit that assumes final medical responsibility for all pregnancies, births, and newborns in its many-county region.

A network of such centers, each housed in a long-existing general hospital, blankets the state. Each prenatal office visit, each step of prenatal care, and the current status of each patient is registered on a coded computer card with the regional center.

By the early 1980s, predicts Dr. Jack M. Schneider, pregnancies could be similarly monitored nationwide. Then virtually every fetus nestled or kicking in every womb throughout America would have an electronic guardian angel in the form of a watchful computer.

Thus, when Jennie Eagle's record shows a history of diabetes in her family, the computer will print out a letter to remind her doctor that a test for abnormal glucose tolerance should be employed to check Jennie for the disease. When a routine blood test on Mona Henney indicates a rare metabolic disorder, the computer will suggest she be referred to the regional center for special tests and possible application of a new remedy. And when Jean Tabor unexpectedly gives birth while on vacation in Boston, her small pelvic measurement and tendency to bleed easily won't surprise her attending physician. Her complete medical picture and prenatal course of treatment, with danger signs asterisked, sent from her regional center by telephone lines, will be printed out in the delivery suite.

Backing up the computers will be live obstetric consultants who will confer by phone with patients' physicians in complicated cases, while following up on computer warnings of possible errors or omissions in individual treatment.

This medical dream of the future doesn't sound implausible in Wisconsin, where much of the framework to make it possible has already been constructed. Indeed Wisconsin, more than any other state, is a showcase of regional perinatal care, a concept recommended for the future by national physicians' organizations and governmental agencies alike. And the program has been planned and put into action in

Wisconsin not with massive Federal or foundation grants and direction, but with state and local funding, through the initiative and cooperation of doctors, nurses, and hospital administrations.

Seven regional perinatal centers have now been established throughout the state, so that 90 percent of Wisconsin's population is within an hour's drive of a center and no resident is more than two and one-half hours away from one. Joined by common interests, nurtured by the state's two medical schools, linked by a Wisconsin Perinatal Association, the centers are nevertheless each independent and locally led.

All of the centers have unmet goals. All are in various stages of growth, ranging from the newest, at Neenah, which began in late 1971 with a newborn intensive-care unit, to the oldest, established in Madison and Milwaukee in 1968 and 1969. The latter centers, both university-based, offer a wide range of facilities and services to patients and doctors in their regions, and highly specialized services to patients and staff of the other centers.

In 1974 the Madison center will add its pilot project of computer-monitored prenatal care, which it hopes all other centers will adopt. By 1975 every medically known pregnancy in Madison and the fourteen counties surrounding it, an area encompassing twenty-eight hospitals and 13,000 births annually, will probably be so monitored.

The success of the centers is proved daily in terms of life and death. Thus, the new center in the Mississippi River town of La Crosse (population 50,000) in its first year dropped the newborn mortality rate in its nine-county region from the national average of 16 per thousand live births to 9.2 per thousand.

The Milwaukee center, based at Milwaukee County

Hospital, in a few years has halved newborn mortality in its region. Amazingly, it has reduced newborn mortality among Milwaukee's low-income population—blacks, Indians, poor whites—all served by County, to below the level of the rest of Milwaukee, which is about the national average.

In the prosperous south-central Wisconsin block of counties served by the center at Madison, newborn mortality has plunged since 1967 from 15 per thousand live births to below 8. Some time before the end of 1974, estimates Stanley N. Graven, M.D., professor of pediatrics, University of Wisconsin Medical School, neonatologist and codirector of the perinatal center at Madison, that figure will have dropped to a near-irreducible 4.0 or 5.0.

It was Stanley Graven who pioneered the idea of regional perinatal care in Wisconsin. Brought to Wisconsin by the University of Wisconsin and located in Madison's St. Mary's Hospital in 1966 to establish a newborn program, he was named by the Wisconsin Academy of Pediatrics to head a statewide study of premature births, stillbirths, and newborn deaths.

In the study, which covered all such cases in thirty-five Wisconsin hospitals for a three-year period, he found that "about one-third of the deaths were clearly nonpreventable—drastic congenital defects, that sort of thing. One-third were preventable locally if they had just applied existing knowledge, simple techniques—things like body temperature, adequate administration of oxygen, resuscitating the baby adequately, feeding him properly, recognizing that the baby was either infected or jaundiced or had disease for which he should have been treated.

"Another third of the deaths were difficult cases but could have been prevented if you had had a team of trained people with adequate resources. An example would be a small premature baby with respiratory distress. You would need a team. You would need a pediatrician, a respirator with somebody who knows how to operate it, a blood-gas laboratory and a blood bank with technicians on hand around the clock, a good radiologist, specially trained nurses, all working together. That meant a center, because no one hospital had enough cases to support such a team.

"So this means that in America during those recent years, when we were losing nationwide about sixteen to eighteen newborns per thousand, more than many other nations, and in Wisconsin were losing about fifteen per thousand, four to six were nonpreventable, four to six should have been prevented locally—no excuse for them—and four to six were pretty tough problems but still clearly preventable.

"The fetal deaths [stillbirths of enough maturity—twenty-six weeks or more—to survive had they been born alive] broke out about the same way. Out of twelve per thousand live births, one-third to one-half were nonpreventable, one-fourth to one-third were preventable if attended by a center, one-third were preventable with proper care locally.

"So on the basis of that study," explained Dr. Graven, "we set about organizing regional centers."

This was something different than was occurring elsewhere in America. Medical schools throughout the land were vying to establish sophisticated medical units to care for high-risk pregnancies and critically ill newborns. Beginning in the late 1950s, the new medical sciences of fetology (study and care of the fetus) and neonatology (study and care of the newborn) had made rapid advances, and a handful of working units had already been established. But little or no effort was expended by the new centers in improving care beyond their walls.

"Ultimately," explained Stanley Graven, "if the center was going to do its job, it not only had to provide complex care in the center. It had to go out to every community hospital and see that those four or five locally preventable deaths didn't occur either.

"In the long run, we do more to improve health care for mothers and babies by what we do out there than by what we do here. If we do our job right, out there, we'll ultimately have half as many babies coming here. We'd like nothing better than to make newborn intensive care unnecessary."

Once the survey results were in, the most crucial task began: persuading doctors and nurses to change their ways, to upgrade care.

The campaign is still spoken of wonderingly by those who saw it in action: Stanley Graven, the "young whippersnapper" trying to teach the old dogs new tricks. His partner on the sawdust trail, was Helen Callon, R.N., the grand old lady of Wisconsin nursing, nursing consultant for maternal-child health in the state department of health, his bridge to the state's nurses and his guide in avoiding the reefs and shoals of local medical politics.

"We organized annual one-day teaching sessions," recalls Stanley Graven, "in eight or ten places throughout the state. Each year we'd reach eight hundred to one thousand nurses, and a lot of doctors."

But at first only a handful of physicians came, because many objected to being educated in company with nurses, as peers. Once the nurses started coming home "educated beyond the doctors," as Helen Callon put it, the doctors' resistance crumbled.

In addition to the one-day institutes, Graven's task

force inaugurated a program in which hospitals, by request, were analyzed and given recommendations by a visiting team of physicians and nurses. In its first three years of operation, the program surveyed eighty hospitals.

"We just sort of preached the message," Graven told me, "of good early care for babies, attention to detail, looking for problems, understanding what you're looking for, how to give oxygen, how to keep babies' temperatures up, how to feed them properly. . . . Finally, we told them how to create a perinatal center. . . . If you think you've got troubles, call the center. . . . If the baby's got troubles, call the center. The center will come and get him.

"So 1969 was the first full calendar year that the newborn center in Madison operated. We started in July 1968 with our neonatal intensive-care unit. And in February of 1969 Milwaukee County Hospital opened theirs. The next ones opened in early 1970—La Crosse, Marshfield, and Green Bay. Neenah opened theirs in October of 1971, and Dubuque across the Mississippi in Iowa, in early 1972."

Proof of success was fast in coming. For example, twenty-one small hospitals (staffed entirely by general practitioners) that referred difficult cases to the Madison center experienced a drop in newborn mortality from 14.2 per thousand in 1965–1966 to 7.7 in 1969. The large hospitals in the region, staffed by specialists, failed to refer babies to or use the center in 1969. And their newborn mortality rate dropped only from 15.6 to 13.8 during the same period.

"Thus," explained Stanley Graven, "in 1969 if you were a mother who delivered a premature baby, your baby's chances for survival were best if you were cared for by a general practitioner out in a small town. Because you didn't get caught in medical politics. You didn't get caught in the professional ego of the specialist who wasn't able to do as well for that baby as the center was. And this of course was very devastating to professional egos."

But by 1970 virtually all critically ill newborns in Madison were being referred to the regional newborn unit. And the Madison newborn mortality rate had dipped to eight per thousand.

So far, a regional perinatal center did not really exist at Madison, only a newborn intensive-care unit with a strong commitment to education. But in 1971 the parts of what would be the perinatal center started coming together. The University of Wisconsin Medical School closed its newborn and obstetrics wards in University Hospital and placed its fetal-perinatal faculty in charge of births and newborns in two Madison hospitals a few blocks away from each other: St. Mary's, site of Graven's unit, and Madison General. Of 4600 annual births in Madison, all but 400 now occur in the joined St. Mary's–Madison General facility; someday all of them may.

Ideally, a regional perinatal center has everything close together: a weekly prenatal clinic for high-risk pregnancies, an intensive-care maternity ward, an intensive-care unit for newborns, round-the-clock blood bank and laboratories for infant blood-gas studies, blood typing, radiology. Plus a wide range of medical specialists on call for consultation, treatment, and surgery, and specially trained nurses and M.D.s on duty at all times. Plus much more, including fetal and infant monitoring equipment. And all guided by a troika superskilled in perinatal medicine: an obstetrician-fetologist, a neonatologist to watch the newborns, and a perinatal nurse to develop and guide the crucially important nursing care.

Madison has all of these, spiritually one though under three roofs: Madison General Hospital, site of the high-risk obstetric care unit; St. Mary's, site of high-risk newborn care; and University Hospital, workplace of internists, cardiac surgeons, and other University nonperinatal specialists. Though inconvenient at times, it is obviously working as a pragmatic solution to what seemed an insoluble problem in medical politics.

Still, in 1972 when it was finally all together, much remained to be done. This was especially true for the obstetrical half of the perinatal center. For while newborn mortality rates had been plunging downward in areas of the state served by newborn intensive-care centers, stillbirths remained at twelve per thousand, the rate of five and ten years before. Care of the unborn and their mothers had not changed enough to save the one-half to two-thirds of stillbirths which by Graven's calculations were preventable.

Dr. Jack M. Schneider, the codirector of the Madison perinatal center, explained to me that the solution, as in newborn care, would have to come from an outreach by the university, through the regional centers.

"We're saying that the major, important thing for a center, in its own region, is to continually sponsor education programs, to retread the old tires and keep the new tires from wearing down. And so we of the university help regional centers sponsor institutes around the state. We hold quarterly conferences here at Madison, as do other regional centers. The Madison center, at the direction of the Wisconsin Perinatal Association, publishes a monthly newsletter carrying basic information on recent developments in prenatal and newborn care, and sends it to every physician in the state who delivers babies, to every hospital nursery, and to many doctors and hospitals in nearby Great Plains states.

"We're trying to create a unit that will have some relation with the outside world. That's different. Most university centers are totally cloistered into themselves. They teach exemplary medicine. But the medical students go out and discover that what the medical school teaches they can't do. They're trained to rely on specialists. If it's heart trouble, you call Charlie. If it's an ingrown toenail, talk to Clyde. Then they get their M.D. degree and set up practice in northwestern Wisconsin and they're all those nine specialists!

"So large regions of the United States have general practitioners who are marginal people, not because they're generalists but because they're trained to have specialist consultative backup and then all of a sudden they're in an environment where it's not available."

The situation in metropolitan regions in some ways is even worse, according to Dr. Schneider. "In cities, there is probably less referral and consultation. Big-city folks tend to be more self-assured about their competence. They're more worried about their prestige. And they're afraid to refer the patient for fear they'll lose her forever to the specialist. (Something the fellow one hundred miles away doesn't have to worry about.)"

The new M.D. with a big obstetrical problem on his hands may try to get help from a typical university center—once or twice. He soon learns better. "Here's this man in private practice working eighteen hours a day," explains Dr. Schneider. "He has a patient five months along and at seven P.M. she's starting to go into labor. He calls the university medical center and explains the whole thing to an intern, or a nurse, who finally says, 'Yeah, we'd better have Dr. Whiz call you.' They go looking for him, which takes six hours. Dr. Whiz doesn't call back until the next day. And when he calls back, he tells the family doctor about all this exciting research stuff that he and his colleagues have done in goats and sheep."

In Wisconsin today, any physician can pick up the phone night or day and get immediate consultation in obstetrics from Dr. Schneider or one of his two associates, who on off-hours are always within reach by radiophone. Another similar hot line puts a doctor in touch with the chief of service of newborn intensive care, for immediate advice on treating or transferring to the center a critically ill newborn.

At least 10 percent of obstetric patients, on the average, fall into the category of extreme high risk and therefore are expected to benefit from consultative management and sometimes delivery at a regional perinatal center. A main thrust of perinatal education for doctors in Wisconsin is to get them to separate high risks from normals and give the high risks more than routine attention.

"Some losses are inevitable, even with the best of care in the best possible regional center," says Dr. Schneider. "But a doctor shouldn't lose a baby because he is delivering a severe diabetic mother in a thirty-bed hospital; her baby can be expected to be in trouble at birth and need special care. He shouldn't lose an Rh baby as a stillbirth because he didn't do an amniocentesis. He shouldn't lose a baby to infection because he waited thirty-six hours to get it delivered."

An important way to decrease stillbirths in Wisconsin and elsewhere, believes Dr. Schneider, will be to increase the knowledge and techniques of nurses who staff delivery suites.

"As soon as you leave the centers with full-time house staff, the nurse is the one who delivers the obstetrical care around the time of birth," says Schneider.

"Visit hospital maternity wards across the United States and in each one you'll find a file containing three-by-five-inch cards."

"The cards," adds Beverly Aure, R.N., coordinator of nursing at the perinatal center in Madison, "are called 'routine obstetrical orders,' which means that every patient is the same. Well, they aren't the same. On the card is how much medication to give any patient if she's dilated so much. The card is a contract between nurse and doctor that if nothing is really wrong the nurse will follow the case."

"And," says Dr. Schneider, "the card also tells the nurse when the doctor wants to be called. There are a few doctors who want to be called on every case, right away. Some specify, 'No calls eleven P.M. to seven A.M.' But the feeling of the vast majority of doctors is, "Get me there on time, don't embarrass me, but don't get me there too early. And don't bother me too much before. If you bother me, be sure it's something urgent because I'm a busy, tired guy and I have higher priorities than obstetrics—my office practice, or gynecological surgery.'

"So the nurses are delivering the intrapartum care —the care during labor and delivery—while the doctor sees patients in his office or gets a few more winks of sleep. And in virtually all American hospitals, nurses have not been formally trained to do this."

"They would like to be," says Ms. Aure. "It's obvious at our conferences and hospital visits how eager they are to soak up the knowledge that will help them determine priorities of care and give substance to their intuitive experience."

To understand how regional perinatal care works today in Wisconsin and can work tomorrow in every area, consider a recent case:

Mrs. Betty O., twenty-three, of Beloit, Wisconsin, breezed uneventfully through her first pregnancy despite the fact that a valve in her heart had been damaged by rheumatic fever.

But three months later, real trouble of another kind developed. Mrs. O. began to suffer from lupus erythematosus, a connective-tissue disease that is life-threatening when it involves the kidneys. Hers did. She lay for three months in a bed in University Hospital in Madison, while hot and cold packs were applied to her swollen joints and hurting chest, and powerful drugs fought her disease. Finally the attack subsided and she returned home, apparently back to normal but still taking azathioprine to guard against rheumatic fever and cortisone to counter lupus erythematosus.

She needed strength to run her busy household. For, in addition to the baby, she cared for six stepchildren, ages six to fifteen.

The following summer the family moved from Beloit to Kenosha in southeastern Wisconsin, and Betty O. discovered that she was pregnant again.

Mrs. O. could have found a family physician in Kenosha who would have provided basic medical attention, with the regional perinatal center in Madison providing specialized care. Regional centers prefer to work this way whenever possible, especially so that they won't be accused of stealing patients from private physicians.

But Mrs. O. knew that hers was a high-risk pregnancy. With her chronic diseases, she suspected she would require special care. She became a patient of the high-risk clinic of the Wisconsin Perinatal Center in Madison, with Dr. Jack Schneider as her primary physician.

The high-risk clinic, held twice weekly in the outpatient area of Madison General Hospital, coordinated all aspects of Betty O.'s care. The medication for her chronic diseases continued under the supervision of her "kidney doctor," renal specialist Lawrence R. Hyman, M.D., of the University of Wisconsin Medical School. A dietitian outlined an appropriate diet. An ultrasonic technician made sonar "pictures" of her unborn baby. Any resource of the hospital or university could be tapped quickly to help her, including, if necessary, the services of a psychologist or social worker.

Dr. Schneider prescribed antibiotics to counter a recurrent bacterial infection of the urinary tract, present in more than 5 percent of all pregnancies and potentially dangerous to the mother and fetus. Because Betty O. had had rheumatic fever damage, he made a note to give antibiotics during labor, delivery, and in the days following birth, to prevent reinfection of the heart during this stressful time. And after birth, her Fallopian tubes would be tied to prevent the great danger that would be posed by any future pregnancy.

A major hazard facing Betty O. and her unborn baby was toxemia, which affects one in twenty pregnant American women and is a leading cause of infant and maternal illness and death.

Lupus erythematosus may damage the kidneys even more during pregnancy, in which case the mother's kidneys would not be able to excrete all the wastes of mother and baby, especially during the latter third of pregnancy. This could precipitate toxemia, with harmful results that can include swollen limbs, high blood pressure, convulsions, and coma.

In Betty O.'s case, Dr. Schneider decided to head off the possibility of toxemia or intrauterine death by delivering the baby early, as soon as it could survive well outside its mother's body.

But how mature was he? His date of conception was

unknown. If delivered too late he might suffer from toxemia, but if delivered before his lungs were mature enough (a point usually reached at about thirty-five weeks' gestation), he could develop hyaline membrane disease.

Shortly after Christmas, Dr. Schneider told Betty O. that it was almost time to deliver the baby. A test of fluid taken from the amniotic sac around the baby revealed the presence of an adequate amount of surfactant in the baby's lungs.

But nature beat the doctors to the draw. Just before midnight, January 2, Mrs. O. began having labor pains. Her husband bundled her up, and, with her sister's husband driving, they hurried toward Madison General Hospital 110 miles away. (Somewhat farther than any patient should be from a regional center. Eventually, it is planned, there will be a regional perinatal center serving the Kenosha-Racine area.)

On the outskirts of Madison the car blew a tire, and Mrs. O.'s "bag of water" broke. Contractions were coming three minutes apart. The O.'s arrived at the hospital at 1:30 A.M. and at 1:59 A.M. a healthy six-pound son was born. A week later, without complications, mother and baby joined the family at home.

Had the birth been induced, as planned, it would not have been so dramatic. But additional facilities of the regional perinatal center would have swung into action. The sequence would go like this:

Betty O. checks into Madison General Hospital for induced labor and delivery in the maternal intensive-care unit of the hospital's obstetrics ward, a component of the regional perinatal center. She meets her attending physician, who begins the induction by means of intravenous infusion of the labor-stimulant drug, oxytocin.

Instead of being under the care of a general nurse trained "on the job" in obstetrics care, she is overseen by a perinatal nurse specialist, a new kind of nurse with a master's degree in high-risk perinatal nursing. The nurse directly giving her care may be the specialist or a nurse-clinician, an R.N. with one or more years of obstetric nursing experience, who has been university-trained for several months in the new perinatal discipline. The latter knows what symptoms to watch for, what to do when they get out of hand, and when to call in a doctor. (In fact, she has more obstetric training than a family doctor.) She is able to read and interpret the electronic fetal monitor, which is employed in every high-risk birth at a regional perinatal center. And she keeps an eye on the delicate automatic infusion pump that drips labor stimulant into Mrs. O.'s body at a preset rate. The fetal monitor may reveal that the labor stimulant is working too well, causing prolonged contractions that threaten the baby. Then the labor stimulant flow is decreased or stopped. In addition, a sample of blood may be taken from the scalp of the unborn baby, and analyzed to assess the fetal condition.

A staff M.D. checks repeatedly with Mrs. O. and her nurse-clinician. In a true regional perinatal center, an obstetrician is continuously on hand around the clock to manage high-risk labor and delivery. At a university-based regional center, this is the chief resident physician and almost always the obstetric codirector of the perinatal center. So when Mrs. O. finally delivers, she does so not just in the company of one doctor and one nurse—standard staffing at the average American delivery.

In addition, Mrs. O.'s nurse-clinician is present to watch both patients—the one outside and the one inside; the fetal monitor has been wheeled into the delivery room still wired into the mother.

Also present is a perinatal anesthesiologist, especially trained in administering pain relief during birth in such a way that Mrs. O.'s damaged heart and kidneys can withstand the strain. Even more crucial is his task of guarding the unborn baby, of preventing the anesthetic or a pinched umbilical cord from starving his brain of oxygen. Because high-risk mothers frequently give birth to high-risk infants, he must be ready to aid in the resuscitation of the baby immediately at the time of birth.

Still another M.D.—a neonatologist—is present in the delivery room to assess the baby's condition, to suction his breathing passages and perhaps pump oxygen into his lungs, and, if necessary, to place him in a waiting, prewarmed incubator and rush him into the newborn intensive-care unit of the perinatal center.

Once in the newborn intensive-care unit, which is the more elaborate, complex, and costly wing of any perinatal center, the ill baby has much more than a fighting chance. Here, under the medical management of a neonatologist and the nursing management of a clinical nurse specialist, he is guarded minute by minute by the kind of superskilled nursing attention and equipment described in Chapter VIII. He is fed intravenously and tapped for blood samples through a catheter that remains inserted in his umbilical cord. His breathing, temperature, oxygen intake, and heartbeat are monitored electronically. An M.D. is always on hand.

He may weigh only three pounds—or two. His heart may stop, or his breathing; but immediately an alarm rings and a nurse restarts the motion. A laboratory and a blood supply are available twenty-four hours a day to serve him. If necessary, a machine will breathe for him.

Not only does he now have a good chance for life, but a far better chance of growing up undamaged mentally or physically than if the perinatal center did not exist.

The resources of a university medical center are rich. They are also rare and costly, largely funded by research grants and education monies.

What kind of a regional perinatal center can be established in a non-university setting?

To find out, leave Madison and travel west over green rolling hills, past wooded bluffs and streams, fields of corn and tobacco, and neat dairy farms to the bustling Mississippi River town of La Crosse.

Meet young Dr. Mike Hartigan, a pediatrician in private group practice at the Gunderson Clinic and codirector of the La Crosse regional perinatal center. Dr. Hartigan shares responsibilities with codirector Jim Tankersley, M.D., who like Hartigan had special training in neonatology before he completed his medical training, and with four of the other nine pediatricians in La Crosse. The six men are alternately on call at the ten- to seventeen-bed neonatal intensive-care unit, which is housed in St. Francis Hospital, one of two hospitals in town. On the day of my visit, there are nine tiny babies in the unit. Each wears a tiny stocking nightcap. The younger and smaller ones, ranging down to two and one-half pounds, are attached to intravenous lines and monitors. Five nurses keep watch over all, while another adjusts the face mask of a respirator pumping air forcefully in and out of a pair of tiny lungs.

"After two and a half years of operation," says Hartigan, "we're getting about ninety percent of the critically ill babies in our region—which includes not only nine Wisconsin counties but three counties in Minnesota and two counties in Iowa. We can handle all but the occasional case, of, say, an unusual metabolic problem that requires all kinds of tests of blood chemistry. Then we send the baby to Madison."

The neonatal unit has laboratory facilities available around the clock. If a baby needs a blood transfusion, as some do every other day, a nurse taps a "walking donor"—a member of the hospital staff already blood-typed and cross-matched for this purpose. (A three-pound premature may only need one-half ounce.)

The university center in Madison provides laboratory and educational backup. Hartigan and his fellow physicians and nurses working with the neonatal unit travel to Madison for conferences and visits, and the Madison center assists the La Crosse center with its programs to educate nurses and doctors of area hospitals about newborn care.

In its first two full years of operation, says Mike Hartigan, the unit lowered newborn mortality in the region from 16 deaths per thousand live births to 9.7.

So far, at this visit, the obstetrical half of the perinatal unit was only in the planning stages.

"Obstetrics in this town is very sophisticated," explains Dr. Hartigan. "But they just don't happen to want to put it all together."

Hartigan suggests that consolidation of obstetric and pediatric services would offer better utilization of space, personnel, and equipment.

He's working with local obstetricians to persuade them to accept an educational commitment for all doctors who deliver babies in the region.

"The specialists," says Hartigan, "have a responsibility not only to handle the complicated perinatal problems that are referred to them. They also have a responsibility to keep referring physicians abreast of good care so they know which patients to refer and how to take superb care of the patients they keep.

"If we don't do this on our own—this is one thing I'm sure of—it will come painfully from an outside source—either statewide or from the Federal Government—which can almost be guaranteed to make an inaccurate assessment of the situation and levy some laws that may or may not have pertinence.

"Of all the babies we've 'rescued,' the case that most sticks in my mind began at two o'clock in the morning, a year ago, with a telephone call from a doctor eighty-five miles away in a country town. We were there at three thirty with a doctor, a nurse, an incubator, and an ambulance. A preemie less than three pounds who's done beautifully. Not a particularly difficult case for us. But this doctor was so overwhelmed—not by the care we gave but that after all these years, finally, when he was alone out in the sticks at two o'clock in the morning with a patient in trouble, somebody else cared."

From La Crosse to metropolitan Milwaukee is a giant jump—from the western to the eastern boundary of the state, from a basically rural, healthy area to a big city with a sizable impoverished inner city population. That group is served mainly by Milwaukee County Hospital.

Huge, modern, attractively set in parklike grounds on the western edge of the city, County does not ostensibly fit the welfare hospital image.

"Half of our mothers are clearly high risk," says bearded John Grausz, M.D., a native of Hungary who grew up in Australia, obtained his pediatric boards certification at Yale, and trained in neonatology in

England. For five years, as chief neonatologist, he has directed the evolving perinatal center here. "Two-thirds of our mothers are black. Most, black and white and the rest, are poor, many on welfare.

"This hospital over the years, with fourteen hundred to fifteen hundred births a year, has consistently run thirteen to fifteen percent low birthweight. So one might expect our mortality rate to be more than double the rate of other hospitals in the community that serve the prosperous population, and whose rate is about the national average. In fact, we have the lowest mortality rate, even though we also are referred many of the most difficult obstetric cases in the city, from all income levels."

Why is the inner city population in Milwaukee high risk?

"Because it's a poor group, with many different kinds of problems. They don't seek prenatal care with the same diligence as the middle-class person. It's hard to get them to the clinic even if they know they are diabetic or whatever; they may go their way and turn up with a dead fetus six months later.

"They have a toxemia rate that's close to fifteen percent, whereas the rate for private middle-class patients is two to three percent. And this has to do, largely, with lack of prenatal care."

Is malnutrition a major factor?

"I suspect," answers Grausz, "that there is some nutritional deprivation, but not malnutrition that you can detect physiologically—aside from obesity, which is frequent.

"Many mothers are very young unwed teen-agers; it's a poor time of life to have a baby. They may try to hide the pregnancy. They face possible rejection at home and in school.

"Many of the mothers are older than the norm, and have had several children, which makes them high risk.

"There's a lot of preexisting illness and damage from previous illness in the mothers. Not rickets so much now. But we get some spinal problems that make a mother's respiration difficult. We have sickle-cell anemia problems in black mothers."

County Hospital is only one of sixteen hospitals in the Milwaukee area that deliver babies, and it does not deliver the largest number. But it contains the only full-blown perinatal center in the city, staffed by full-time obstetricians, pediatricians, and other M.D.s—all on the faculty of the private Medical College of Wisconsin. St. Luke's Hospital, which serves the southern half of the city, has started to develop a perinatal center, as have two other hospitals.

In the future, Dr. Grausz would like to see all births in Milwaukee taking place at two or three centers. "But I don't expect to see it happening in my lifetime," he sighs.

Still, "we get good referrals for high-risk newborns, and are in the process of working through the problems of where high-risk mothers should be delivered. There must be rules that only fully staffed and equipped hospitals like this should handle certain kinds of high-risk cases."

In five years, Grausz and his staff have more than halved the mortality and illness rates of babies born in the hospital. Those born at the hospital who have to go to the thirty-five-bed intensive-care unit are usually soon "graduated" because they have received top care from birth.

"Our little babies don't get severe hyaline membrane disease," says Grausz. "Of two hundred premature births annually in the hospital, only four or five have severe hyaline membrane disease—and they recover from it unless they have other problems."

Showing a visitor about his nursery, which that day contains twenty-nine babies, Dr. Grausz points out four frail newborns that each weigh less than two pounds.

"We just had a visitor from Germany who stated categorically that babies under fifteen hundred grams [3.3 pounds] don't survive. In his hospital they don't even try to save them.

"Our survival rate for *two-pounders*—who do not have bleeding, who get here in good shape—is by and large about ninety percent. For all babies of this weight it's an eighty-five-percent survival rate, with probably better than seventy-five percent physically and mentally intact. We see them later, at two and three years, and they are a pleasure—'Sesame Street' students, some of whom can count to ten and spell out words."

Back in Madison, Dr. Stanley Graven discusses the lesson of Milwaukee as it relates to perinatal care in America.

"The medical community has long taken the position that our high U.S. infant mortality rate has been due primarily to our socioeconomic conditions. That's garbage. That's a smoke screen. Create the illusion that our problems are created by the people, not by the inadequacies of the health-care delivery system.

"What our studies show is that there are things that need to be done socially. We aren't negating that. The fact that you've got poor socioeconomic conditions simply means that you've got more to deliver with more care. This John Grausz has shown: Milwaukee County Hospital serves the poorest population in the state, in terms of socioeconomic conditions. Yet this hospital has the lowest mortality rate of any hospital in the city. And that's because of care. County gives the best care.

"This doesn't mean that the man in general pediatric or obstetric practice isn't competent. It just means that if he wants to be comparably competent, he has to be *here*. You can't have facts funneled to you over the phone. You can't run back and forth from office practice to hospital and end up with the same level of competence in terms of the care delivered.

"We say that the doctor and the nurse ought to be standing *together* beside the patient to decide what they see, and what that means and what they together ought to do about it. That is the only way to make decisions of this magnitude."

Today Drs. Stanley Graven, Jack Schneider, John Grausz, Mike Hartigan, R.N.s Helen Callon, Beverly Aure, and their colleagues have dreams that extend far beyond the borders of Wisconsin.

The dreams are embodied in The Great Plains Organization for Perinatal Care, which is designed to spread Wisconsin-type perinatal care networks across the entire breadth of the Dakotas, Nebraska, Minnesota, and Iowa, in addition to Wisconsin. State perinatal societies, each composed of neonatologists, fetologists, obstetricians, pediatricians, family physicians, nurses, and other health professionals, are beginning to trade information, cooperate in joint training programs and conferences, and help each other campaign for legislative support of the perinatal idea. In 1973 the membership included representatives from seventeen perinatal centers in various stages of development.

As odd as it may seem to a professor of medicine at

Harvard or a native of Manhattan, the most extensive and advanced model of regional perinatal care in the United States is now evolving in the cornfields of the Midwest. As it prospers, so will the chances for similar care for every mother-to-be and unborn child in America.

CHAPTER

XIII

When Mothers in Labor Need Help: Cesareans and Induced Births

Obstetrics' most dramatic moments come in life-and-death situations when nature seems to have failed. Then the doctor must step in as rescuer to get the baby out before it's too late.

The drama may be played out in tense weeks of waiting for an ill unborn to mature enough to survive in the outside world. When tests reveal it is ready, birth is induced by gradual infusion into the mother's bloodstream of oxytocin.

Or the drama may be a race of minutes between the surgeon's knife and extinction of an unborn life, in an emergency Cesarean section. At such a time, says a physician, "tension fills the operating room like hot gas in a nonexpanding balloon."

For answers to questions about the two methods of "artificial birth"—Cesarean section and induced labor —I interviewed Gerald G. Anderson, M.D., chief of obstetrics at Yale–New Haven Medical School. In addition, I sought answers from three physicians at the University of Southern California Medical School: Dr. Edward Quilligan, head of the department of obstetrics and gynecology; Dr. Roger Freeman, chief of obstetrics; and Dr. Edward Hon, chief of the section of perinatal biology and prime authority on electronic fetal monitoring. ("A" in Q and A stands for Anderson; other interviewees are fully named.)

Q. How often are births artificially induced?

A. At some hospitals, the figure runs up to 20 percent. Here, at Yale–New Haven Medical Center, it's about 10 percent.

Q. On what occasions do you induce labor?

A. We do it usually because of some underlying disease in the mother that adversely affects the fetus. For example, diabetes in the mother frequently causes the baby to die in utero, in the last trimester. Or Rh disease. Or placental insufficiency, in which the baby no longer keeps growing, because it isn't getting enough nourishment from the mother.

If the baby isn't growing, it's really not gaining anything in utero. So then, as in the case of the diabetic or the Rh mother, amniotic fluid is tested for the presence of surfactant as an indication of lung maturity. If the test is positive, we deliver the baby even if it weighs only three pounds.

Another reason to induce would be because the mother lives far from the hospital. Perhaps she lives forty miles from here and had her last child in two hours. When she gets ready, we will induce her just so that she will have the baby in the hospital and not en route in the car.

Q. Are drugs always used to induce birth? Or is it done sometimes solely by breaking the amniotic sac? How often does this latter method work?

A. In a patient who on examination feels "ready" for delivery, rupture of the sac usually results in labor and delivery.

Q. How accurate is the lung surfactant test in determining fetal maturity?

A. We haven't had any errors yet, and we've been doing it more than four years. Some mistakes have been made, and it's mainly because they got a little blood mixed in with the amniotic fluid.

Q. The test originated here at Yale, didn't it?

A. Yes. Dr. Louis Gluck, now the neonatologist at the University of California at San Diego was testing lung surfactant in newborn infants to predict RDS [hyaline membrane disease] due to lung immaturity. We knew that part of the amniotic fluid originated in the lungs, and therefore suggested we test amniotic fluid for the presence of surfactant.

Q. Are there good and bad ways to induce birth? For example, what about the use of injections of birth stimulant (instead of intravenous infusions) still employed at some hospitals? If this suddenly stimulates the mother to have very strong and long contractions endangering the baby, there's no way to modulate the injected oxytocin, is there?

A. That's absolutely right. Injections should be banned by law. Oral administration of oxytocin, by means of linguettes under the tongue, is also not very precise and has mostly gone out of the picture too.

Q. How should the oxytocin be given?

A. In many hospitals, it is simply dripped into the vein from an IV bottle while a nurse watches the drip rate. This method has a great chance of error. A mechanical device known as an infusion pump provides the ideal means of administering the drug.

Q. Is electronic fetal monitoring necessary during induction?

A. We monitor all inductions—right from the beginning. Without monitoring, you can overstimulate the uterus, make the contractions too long so that the baby is asphyxiated because no oxygen can get through to him. You can give so much that you rupture the uterus. So this has to be watched very, very closely and the monitor is the only way to do it.

DR. HON: Dr. Ronald E. Myers, of the Laboratory of Perinatal Physiology at the National Institutes of Health, has recently published some very significant findings on brain damage he has produced in fetal monkeys, using only oxytocin infusion and anesthesia given to the mother. He produced this damage, including cerebral palsy, by the very techniques that are used worldwide to manage labor! Certainly all induced labor should be monitored. No question about it. No question.

Q. And still, most induced labor is not so monitored?

DR. HON: Most of it is not.

Q. A university obstetrician I've interviewed looks toward the day when most births will be scheduled and induced. Birth, he says, can thus occur precisely at the best time—when the mother is rested and hasn't eaten (a full stomach can be troublesome), when the doctor is rested and all the resources of the hospital are ready and at his command. Amniotic fluid testing, perhaps ultrasound pictures of the baby, and electronic fetal monitoring take away the guesswork. Birth is thus transformed from an emergency procedure—no more mad midnight dashes to the hospital—to something predictable and safer. What do you think of all this; will induced birth someday be preferred over letting nature take its course?

A. Now that we have better ways of diagnosing the fetal condition, of determining fetal maturation, and of monitoring the birth, I think that more and more births will be induced. But as far as a routine thing, just for the heck of it, no.

DR. QUILLIGAN: While we feel you can induce labor very safely, we don't know everything about it, by a long shot. And it's quite possible that there are differences between induced labor and natural labor. Induced labor might not be as good.

Q. How long does induced labor take, as compared with natural labor?

A. About the same time. However, we've done a study here at Yale using prostaglandins rather than oxytocin as a birth stimulant. The prostaglandins were just as safe, and were faster, chiefly because they took effect sooner than did the oxytocin. With groups of easy deliveries, mean delivery time was 5.75 hours with oxytocin and 4.5 hours with prostaglandins.

Q. What happens if you can't induce labor?

A. Then, if there is a medical reason to terminate the pregnancy, we do a Cesarean section.

At approximately this point in the interview, at Yale–New Haven Medical Center, Dr. Anderson was called

away for consultation by an anxious resident. When he
returned, he said:

That was a private patient, having her third baby.
She just arrived at the hospital, they put the electronic monitor on right away and found that the
baby was in trouble. They gave the mother oxygen, and turned her on her side to improve blood
flow to the baby, but it didn't help much. So they
are going to do an emergency Cesarean section on
her right now.

Q. And how quickly will that be done?

A. From right now until the time the baby is out
will be five minutes.

Q. That *fast?*

A. I've taken a baby out in *one* minute, from the
time I picked up the scalpel.

Q. Why such emphasis on speed?

A. Because the baby can survive intact only a few
minutes without oxygen, which happens when
blood isn't getting through the placenta and umbilical cord to the baby. In any case of partial
asphyxia, we never let the baby stay in for more
than half an hour, if we can't completely correct
the condition.

Q. How long does it take for the anesthetic to take
effect?

A. It can be almost immediate—a special crash
induction. We can do this because we have anesthesiologists and obstetricians on duty around the
clock. In smaller units they can't have a setup like
this, and when a patient comes in with a real
emergency, as happened here, they just can't act
very fast. They lose babies.

Q. What would be happening to this baby right
now if the operation were not in progress?

A. He would just get progressively worse and would die, perhaps in half an hour. Or he would have brain damage, would be mentally retarded, or might have cerebral palsy. This case is a good example of fetal monitoring. With a stethoscope, we couldn't have discovered that this baby was in trouble. Although the pattern on the monitor was ominous, the heart rate as detected by stethoscope was in the normal range.

Q. With Hon's pioneering work here, Yale was practically the birthplace of electronic fetal monitoring in the United States. Is it true that you've been able to reduce drastically the number of Cesarean sections because you electronically monitor most births, and thus don't operate on hunches?

A. We have about the same percentage of Cesarean births—about 10 percent—as most places. But now we are sectioning the right patients rather than the wrong ones. In about half of the cases where we used to operate, we no longer do. And we operate on an equivalent number who would not have been sectioned in the old days. All because of electronic fetal monitoring.

Q. Without electronic fetal monitoring, what percentage of Cesareans are unnecessary, would you say?

A. The majority, I am sure. Over 50 percent.

Q. Are there certain benefits from the natural birth process that prepare a baby for life outside —toning up the body, squeezing out fluids, emptying water from the lungs—that a Cesarean baby misses? For example, Dr. Mary Ellen Avery of Montreal Children's Hospital has pointed out that infants delivered by Cesarean section have 20 percent more water in their tissues than babies delivered vaginally.

A. If there is any difference, it's awfully tiny so that it's really insignificant. Cesarean babies are frequently ill, but that is because they were ill even before birth, and that is what made the Cesarean section necessary.

Q. Why is it better for the *mother* to deliver vaginally than by Cesarean?

A. A Cesarean is a major operation. It necessitates the risk of a general anesthetic. There is a risk in any major abdominal surgery—from bleeding, blood clots, other things. Number two, the mother is left with a scar on her uterus; that weakens it. The next time she gets pregnant, the uterus could rupture before she goes into labor, during labor, or actually during the delivery, and rupture carries a very high mortality rate for the mother and the baby. We have to think about how many children the woman wants after this birth. If she's going to have more children, a Cesarean will complicate her life, and she will be sort of an obstetric cripple from that day on.

A Cesarean is inconvenient for her, in that it requires her to be in the hospital for a week or ten days instead of going home with her baby in three days. She can't see her baby for a number of hours after delivery. Breast-feeding is difficult, because the mother is being given morphine to relieve pain, and this keeps her asleep half the time. As with any abdominal surgery, there is pain, and restriction of activity once she arrives home. It takes six weeks for the scar to really heal up well. The extra cost for her and her baby is usually about a thousand dollars.

Q. What about postoperative complications?

A. The uterus is a great big vascular organ, and occasionally after it is sewed up it bleeds internally. You might have to reopen the patient and tie off a vessel. There are a number of complications and it's something that we don't do unless for good reason. Before the antibiotic era—the early 1940s—about five patients per hundred died. But now, with antibiotics, the chief complication of a Cesarean—infection—is gone, so that the risk has been cut way down.

Q. Are there different kinds of Cesarean operation?

A. There is the classical section, which is usually done because it's a very quick procedure. The incision is vertical, on top of the uterus, where it is quite thin, more difficult to repair, more likely to rupture in future pregnancies. If you have more time, you make the incision down at the bottom of the uterus, from one side to the other, where it's easy to repair, and where it's unlikely to rupture.

Q. Does one Cesarean require future Cesareans?

A. A woman who's had a classical Cesarean section normally should have Cesarean deliveries in the future. But if she's had the second type of Cesarean, she is usually delivered vaginally unless the pelvis is too small to deliver the baby.

Q. How long does the second type of Cesarean operation take?

A. It may take ten minutes or so if you are taking your time, from the moment of incision until the baby is out.

Q. How do second and third Cesarean births turn out?

A. Usually the babies turn out very well, in just about the same condition as babies born vaginally. Because this time, it's not an emergency procedure.

Q. Now that we've talked about all the bad things that can happen with a Cesarean, what of the good? When is a Cesarean really valuable and necessary?

A. It's a lifesaving emergency procedure. If the fetal heart rate quickly drops off and it's going down, there's often nothing else we can do. We've got to run in and get the baby out.

And then we have patients who begin labor and are just not progressing, not delivering, no matter what we do. We can't always produce a birth with oxytocin; the success rate is about 85 percent.

If infection has developed in the uterus, a Cesarean operation may be necessary. If the doctor estimates that the labor is going to take, say, twelve hours and you know there is infection in there now, you know you can't wait. If the baby is allowed to remain in that infected amniotic fluid for very long, he can become dangerously infected himself. He'll just have bacteria all through his bloodstream and his lungs. He'll have pneumonia and all sorts of things and may not even live. Sometimes a Cesarean is also done to prevent infection of the baby as he comes down the birth canal, when tests reveal the mother has a dangerous vaginal infection—such as herpes.

DR. FREEMAN: We're very concerned about breech babies. [In a breech birth, which occurs in 3 to 4 percent of all deliveries, the baby comes out backward—buttocks first rather than headfirst, a position that can cause injury to the baby.] We let some deliver vaginally if the delivery progresses well and if it's a good-sized pelvis. But we perform a Cesarean section in 50 to 60 percent of cases where a baby begins to deliver in a breech position. In addition to breech babies, we're also inclined to operate if the baby is too big. We try to section any baby estimated to be larger than nine or nine and a half pounds.

DR. ANDERSON: We tend to do a Cesarean on a breech baby if there is any other complication.

Q. Is a position ever reached when it is impossible to deliver a breech baby?

A. This doesn't happen; the birth just becomes more difficult, harder on the baby. But when a baby comes out headfirst, it dilates the cervix, hour after hour; when the head appears it is fully dilated. Now, it's hard for people to imagine when they look at adults, but in a baby the head is the widest diameter. As the shoulders come through, they are smaller. When the baby delivers buttocks or feet first, the shoulders do the dilating and the head still has to come out; so you have a chance of getting the head stuck in the cervix with the shoulders already out.

Q. Any final remarks about Cesareans or induced births?

Dr. Freeman: When we came to the Los Angeles County–University of Southern California Medical Center in 1970, the Cesarean section rate was low. That's the way I was taught, even as late as 1966. That was—if you can't get something out from below, you've failed. You can drag a lot of things out through the pelvis with a forceps, but I don't think that's using good judgment. But that's the way most of us were trained and that's the way obstetrics is practiced generally in America today.

Obstetrics is just coming out of the dark ages. It's been largely a mechanical art until recently. Diagnosis until recently was very difficult; the fetus was remote. Obstetrics is the last field of medicine to be affected by science.

Delivery by Cesarean section and artificial induction are vitally important parts of modern *precision* obstetrics.

CHAPTER

XIV

Here Come the Supernurses

"It was really an uneasy experience," said the young California housewife. "It was my first pregnancy and I started seeing this doctor who was running a kind of big baby factory. I wanted to ask him about some funny feelings I had, but he seemed so busy. It was 'Hello, you're fine, good-bye.' I felt like I was just another bottle of urine a month to him."

In the years ahead, despite the best intentions of their physicians, more and more pregnant women may get the same feeling. Even with the lowered birth rate, demographers have been predicting an upsurge in births as children of the post-World War II baby boom begin their families. But there will be fewer doctors to deliver those babies. Not only are fewer GPs practicing obstetrics then ever before—63 percent in 1969, for example, as compared with 87 percent in 1959—but also the number of medical students specializing in obstetrics is not increasing and may in fact be declining. And, according to Al Isenman, administrator of the Office of Obstetric-Gynecologic Health Personnel of the American College of Obstetricians and Gynecologists, a continuing problem of maldistribution exists. "There are," he says, "vast areas of the United States without enough obstetricians."

The young California woman switched doctors. And in doing so, she entered an innovative obstetrical care system that appears to be one happy solution to America's abuilding baby-doctor squeeze.

At the Kaiser-Permanente medical center in Bellflower, California, an industrial suburb of Los Angeles, she was first examined and interviewed by obstetrician Kenneth E. Bell, M.D. Her subsequent visits—as long as the pregnancy was entirely normal —alternated between her obstetrician and one of four specially trained nurse practitioners who assist the center's eighteen obstetrician-gynecologists in examining and counseling patients.

When she saw her nurse practitioner, instead of the five-minute visit with her obstetrician—which is the standard time allotment even at Kaiser for a routine prenatal checkup—the new patient was regularly given fifteen minutes, more if she needed it, to ask questions about her mysterious new condition, to voice fears and concerns, to get advice and reassurance from a highly trained and experienced counselor.

Her interviewer was Mrs. Rosalyn Powell, a poised and mellow R.N. who for twenty years, in between rearing her children, has nursed in every area of perinatal care—from labor and delivery rooms to the newborn nursery. In addition, she qualified to become an "obstetric-gynecologic nurse-practitioner" by undergoing a six-month training course given jointly by the obstetrics-gynecology departments of the Kaiser-Permanente Group and the Los Angeles County–

University of Southern California Medical Center. For more than three years, at the Bellflower center, she has been examining and counseling some twenty-four patients a day.

"You build up a closer relationship with the nurse than with a busy doctor," said the pleased new patient. "You feel free to talk and ask questions."

"Women like to talk with women," says Mrs. Powell," and they enjoy bringing up areas and aspects that they are embarrassed to discuss with a man."

Such as?

"Such as things that have sexual connotations in their marital lives. Usually when I first meet an OB patient, I introduce myself and rattle off a range of things that I'm equipped to handle—taking medical history, examining her abdomen, checking the baby's heartbeat, the mother's physical condition, her nutrition, diet, physical activities, travel, sports, sexual activities—I always throw the latter in and invariably that's one of the first things I'm asked about.

"Also, they don't wish to betray their ignorance about their own anatomy to a man. They can ask me about an old wives' tale or bring up some simple question that's been bothering them—like can they raise their hands above their head to dust a shelf. Maybe they'll call me from home, in the middle of housework, with a question like that.

"There's a lot of fear—even after a good childbirth experience. And the hormones of pregnancy cause mood swings, which a husband may not understand, and which can precipitate marital problems. An older married couple may have an unwanted pregnancy. I have the time to listen and to counsel."

Acceptance of the nurses at Bellflower has been enthusiastic. "I have great confidence in the nurse-practitioners," said the new patient. "I always have the feeling that the doctor is there in the background if we need him, if there is any complication. I think the nurse-practitioners know what they're doing—that they're as capable as the doctor in many ways—and that they aren't going to go further than their education and training will allow."

"The patients liked the new system from the beginning," said Lyn Watson, the youngest nurse-practitioner. "I've been doing this two years and I've had only two patients request to see a doctor instead of me. Most say they prefer it over the former system.

"But initially there was a problem of acceptance by the doctors; they were afraid of poor quality health care. We had to prove, before we could practice, that we could catch abnormalities. I don't feel I would miss *anything* gross."

Lyn, a fairly recent R.N. graduate of Cal State, Long Beach, has so far been trained only for gynecologic patient visits—including the annual examination, Pap smear, breast and pelvic exam, history of menstrual irregularities, contraceptive counseling. After further training, she will be able to handle prenatal care.

The training program, a joint project of Kaiser–Permanente and U.S.C., is built in self-contained units or modules so that nurses can begin counseling in specific areas—as Lyn has, in gynecology—before completing all of the training.

"Eventually," says Dr. Kenneth E. Bell, who is director of ob-gyn allied health training for the entire Southern California Permanente Medical Group, which includes twenty nurse-practitioners and seventy-five obstetricians at seven Kaiser medical centers, "it is conceivable that our nurse-practitioners will be given additional training and assist in a broader range of care."

What does that leave for the obstetrician to do?

"Plenty," says Dr. Bell. "Each patient is still followed continually by an assigned obstetrician. Doctors are freed from some of the more routine tasks that nurse-practitioners can do at least as well, and thus have more time for patients with complications, and for study."

The Bellflower group is even finding that nurse-practitioners can increase the quality of care given to complicated cases—who may require extensive counseling, diet advice, or examinations that can be given by the N.P.s.

"Patient satisfaction with this new type of allied health personnel has been extremely gratifying," says Dr. Bell. "In a series of three hundred consecutive postpartum patients, who saw nurse-practitioners prenatally, eighty-five percent felt that with the addition of nurse-practitioners their antepartum care was improved. Only one percent felt that their visits were not instructive. Eighty-five percent said they would like to see a nurse-practitioner during another pregnancy and fifty-two percent went so far as to say that as long as things seemed to be going well they would be willing to see a nurse-practitioner for all of the prenatal visits after their first with a physician."

At this writing, throughout the United States 117 programs for training paramedical personnel in Ob-Gyn were in operation. Of these, 20 to 25 were for nurse practitioners, while 16 were nurse midwife programs. Supernurses are also beginning to appear in hospital maternity wards, taking over functions formerly reserved for doctors. Again, claim proponents, the result is better patient care, akin to the superior care delivered by highly skilled nurses in coronary intensive-care units.

"If small hospitals are going to continue to do obstetrics," says Dr. Ben Peckham, chief of gynecology and obstetrics at the University of Wisconsin, "they are going to have to have round-the-clock coverage by some well-trained people besides doctors—because there aren't enough doctors to deliver such full-time service at hospitals with small maternity services."

The same holds true for larger hospitals in big cities.

"As a student nurse," wrote Mrs. Robert T. Guddee, R.N., in the American Medical Association's *American Medical News*, "I was taught that it was a doctor's duty to do pelvic exams on patients in labor, start intravenous fluids, draw blood, read EKGs, pass nasogastric tubes, and so forth. However, upon moving to San Francisco, I learned to do all these procedures immediately. The doctors do not want to wait until a woman is fully dilated, so they leave that diagnosis to the nurses and wait to be called until the last minute. . . . They often prefer that the nurse decide whether or not to give an additional shot of pain reliever. . . ."

Superskilled obstetrical nurses adequately trained to manage many of these tasks are now evolving, with the blessings of nurses' associations and the American College of Obstetricians and Gynecologists.

Beverly Aure, R.N., tells how supernurses are being utilized at the Wisconsin Perinatal Center, where she is chief of perinatal nursing.

"We've begun with just six—four nurse clinicians and two nurse specialists.

"The nurse clinician, who must be an R.N. and have either a B.S. or one year of obstetrical nursing experience, is the more technically oriented of the two new types of nurses. Her specific responsibility is the technical, physiological, and nursing care of the high-risk obstetrical patient. She knows how to read and interpret the electronic fetal monitor, how to insert the leads for it, how to get fetal scalp samples during delivery. She knows as much as the resident about physiology and disease processes, basic signs and symptoms, lab work, and actually helps to train the new residents. She is never responsible for writing medical orders, yet she is a peer of the resident, and has the added advantage of her nursing knowledge and experience.

"Today nurses are being asked to give opinions and form judgments, and doctors listen—not out of politeness, but because the nurse has something to offer. Then together they form a plan of care. That's different, and the change for many doctors is difficult.

"What we're really trying to establish is that the nurse uses her nursing skill and judgment, and that the doctor need not be responsible for everyone. That nurses are responsible for themselves—if they have the knowledge and do nothing, they are as accountable as the doctor.

"Originally, the nurse-clinician worked only in the labor and delivery rooms. Then, with the opening of our high-risk clinic, we saw an opportunity to improve substantially the continuity of high-risk care: the nurse-clinicians began seeing clinic patients during their prenatal visits. Now, each clinic patient is assigned a nurse-clinician who keeps track of her medical history, makes physical assessments, and really gets to know her patient before she goes into labor. So she gets to know her strengths and limitations, how she copes, and thus is in a position to plan some kind of nursing intervention that will help her get through what may be a difficult situation—not only pregnancy but perhaps a complication with the baby."

The second type of nurse in the Wisconsin center is the nurse specialist. She has a more general, consultative role explains Beverly Aure. In addition to her R.N. degree she has an M.S., broader responsibilities, and is much concerned with human relationships. One function is to act as resource person to the nurse clinician.

One nurse specialist was placed in the special care nursery for ill newborns (ill, but not sick enough for the newborn intensive-care unit). "Her primary task is to upgrade quality of care, keep up with all the latest literature and convey new knowledge to the nursing staff, and also to give support to parents of newborns with special problems—including prematures transferred to the newborn intensive-care unit, babies with mental retardation or congenital deformities."

The second nurse specialist works in the labor and delivery rooms. "Most traditional nurses take good physical care of mothers and babies," Beverly Aure told me, "but they haven't consciously come to grips with the fact that their responsibility is to help people start their families. We're very imbued with this idea, and try to assist both father and mother in their evolving relationship with this new individual in the family. The nurse specialist in the birth rooms has been trying to help obstetrical nurses help the patients more through labor and delivery, and help the fathers give support both in the labor and delivery rooms. If the mother is unwed, we try to make sure that she has some person to support her through labor and delivery—maybe a boy friend (who may be the child's father) or her mother, grandmother, sister. She has as much right to support as anyone else."

The California and Wisconsin experiments prompt the question: if supernurses can successfully take over doctors' tasks in the office and in the hospital, how soon will they take the final step? How soon will they be delivering babies?

They already are. Almost unnoticed for forty years and more, a small group of health professionals has kept alive the tradition of midwifery in North America. In doing so, they have changed their image from that of the ignorant, granny, hills nurse to that of a highly skilled and respected member of the health team. At Yale, Columbia, Johns Hopkins, Kings County Hospital in Brooklyn, and several other leading medical centers, R.N.s undergo an additional year of training to meet a brand-new, soaring demand for qualified nurse-midwives.

Ten years ago, there were fewer than four hundred certified nurse-midwives in the United States. Today there are more than three times as many—still a tiny number, but most official resistance from the medical community has crumbled. In 1970 certified nurse-midwives were endorsed in a joint statement by the American College of Obstetricians and Gynecologists, the Nurses Association of ACOG, and the American College of Nurse-Midwives. The organizations agreed that nurse-midwives, when working under the jurisdiction of a physician, "may assume responsibility for the complete care of the uncomplicated maternity patient."

Dr. Roger Egeberg, while serving as special assistant to the Secretary of HEW in the area of health, referred to nurse-midwives as "urgently needed health-care professionals" and called for legislation to recognize that status. Efforts to permit nurse-mid-wives to practice are under way in several state legislatures. (While at this writing thirty-seven states and jurisdictions permit nurse-midwives to practice, and only two states clearly prohibit them by law, in fifteen states midwives are not permitted to practice due to restrictive interpretation of laws.)

Dr. Sprague Gardiner, 1972–1973 president of the American College of Obstetricians and Gynecologists, recently explained, "Years ago we took delivery away from the midwife to make it a sound scientific specialty. Now the nurse-midwife is part of the team. I think the quality of care for obstetric patients will be augmented rather than diminished."

"In the U.S.," says Eunice K. M. "Kitty" Ernst, R.N., C.N.M., a consultant in nurse-midwifery to the Maternity Center Association of New York City, "we go on the assumption that doctor care across the board is the best, the top. There's a very real question whether this is so—whether a solo doctor can be everything to everybody.

"We feel this is not so. It requires a team—a team that operates laterally, not in a hierarchy—a team in which each person is respected as an individual and as a professional and has an input to make.

"In all of this, nursing has a very important role to play. First of all, because most nurses are women and thus know how women feel. Secondly, because of the way nurses are prepared. They gain an understanding of broad concepts, of the human being as a total entity. The doctor and the nurse should complement one another, not compete."

"In obstetrics, every country in the world other than the U.S. and Canada uses the midwife to care for normal mothers before and during birth. Interestingly, many of these countries have lower infant mortality and morbidity rates than does the U.S.

"No matter how many times we midwives talk to people, they still go back and write about the nurse-midwife without the doctor. They never write about the obstetrical team—the nurse-midwife *and* the doctor *and* the social worker *and* the psychologist and the others.

"The nurse-midwife is one part of the whole thing. I think she could be a very valuable part if we could take the time and make the expenditure to develop nurses in this role. My own impression is that the professional obstetrical nurses we have now, particularly those who hold bachelor's and master's degrees, are wasted if they're not doing midwifery.

"I think most obstetrics nurses would have been midwives if they had been given the opportunity. Most I've talked with deplore the fact that they are constantly being given responsibilities they have not been trained to handle. Sure, they've delivered babies from time to time—and have lost years off their lives by sweating it out. It's one thing to catch a baby and say 'I managed,' and it's another thing to support a mother in the delivery of her child and to feel really good about it—to know that you did a comprehensive job in the light of present obstetrical knowledge."

Kitty Ernst is a prime example of the intelligent, highly educated, modern midwife who promises to play such an important role in today's obstetrical revolution. After securing her R.N., she trained and then practiced as a midwife with the famous Frontier Nursing Service in eastern Kentucky. In a poor, seven-hundred-square-mile mountainous area where doctors are few, the service is a model of rural health care. It owns and runs a twenty-six-bed hospital and outpatient clinic staffed by physicians, but the chief health-care facilities are six nursing outposts scattered over the three-county area. Each station is staffed by two or three nurses and nurse-midwives who furnish some four hundred families with comprehensive health care by means of their own special skills and by following written medical orders and telephone and radio directions from physicians at the central hospital. On many occasions, the nurses and nurse-midwives travel up winding, narrow mountain roads by Jeep—once it was by horseback—to visit families in their homes. In their first 10,000 deliveries, the Frontier nurse-midwives kept their maternal mortality rate to one-third of the national and state levels; during the past twenty years, they have not lost a mother.

After beginning with British-trained nurse-midwives, the Frontier Nursing Service in 1939 established its own graduate school of nurse-midwifery, which has instructed approximately one-third of all U.S.-trained nurse-midwives.

Kitty Ernst left the Frontier Nursing Service to practice in New York City for the Maternity Center Association, founded in 1931 as the first institution in America to provide formal training for midwives. In poor sections of the city, she attended home deliveries (since discontinued). She graduated from Hunter College, earned a master of public health degree from Columbia University School of Public Health and Administrative Medicine, then took charge at Columbia of a master's degree program in nursing that included midwifery. She married, moved to Philadelphia, bore three children, taught parent-preparation classes, took a refresher course in midwifery at Kings County Hospital in Brooklyn, and ended up as a four-day-a-week consultant in midwifery assigned by the Maternity

Center Association of New York to Philadelphia's Booth Maternity Center. The latter is a former Salvation Army home and hospital for unwed mothers-to-be that in 1971 was expanded into a community maternity hospital, serving all social classes. Two obstetricians and a pediatrician direct the medical service, conduct initial examinations of mothers-to-be, and handle complications; one is on hand whenever there is a birth. But four nurse-midwives manage prenatal care and deliveries in all normal pregnancies.

How adequate is the training of the nurse-midwife? Few Americans realize that the modern midwife receives far more training in obstetrics than does the GP. With certain exceptions, her midwifery training is concentrated solely upon pregnancy and childbirth, whereas the GP's training covers the entire range of human disorders. Similarly, though to a somewhat lesser extent, the midwife has certain advantages over the obstetrician-gynecologist, much of whose specialized training has been spent in surgery and gynecology. After graduation, the nurse-midwife accumulates more experience per year in managing normal pregnancies than does the obstetrician-gynecologist, for she spends full time at it, as he does not. (Admittedly, an obstetrician accumulates much more experience in normal deliveries during his three or four years of residency than does the nurse-midwife during her one year of training. However, many nurse-midwives have prior experience in obstetrical nursing.)

The midwife does not use forceps, general anesthesia, nor does she perform Cesarean sections. She can perform an episiotomy, a minor operation to prevent tearing of the vulva during labor, and give local anesthetics as needed.

Her inclination is to let nature take its course so long as everything is normal, whereas pressures upon the doctor tempt him to give nature a shove.

The strong point of the midwife is continuous support of the mother-to-be throughout pregnancy and delivery, which often the doctor cannot provide.

"The midwife," explains Dr. John B. Franklin, chief of staff at Booth Maternity Center, "really gets to know the patient during pregnancy; and she keeps records on the patient's feelings and her expectations of pregnancy. When the patient comes in for labor, she sees a nurse-midwife she has met before. And the contract with this woman is that she's going to get labor support. The midwife does not leave her side; it is a one-to-one relationship. The contract is not that she is going to get labor support without anything else. The midwife is there to see that she is as free from anxiety as possible, as comfortable as possible, and to see that with her husband's help she can cope with her labor.

"Then the doctor's role is placed once again in its traditional framework. He is there to watch for complications. He makes assessments to see if progress is being made, whether there's need for intervention, whether any of his skills are needed—such as giving conduction, caudal, or epidural anesthesia. He does not provide labor support unless there's some conflict —as when the nurse-midwife has to be someplace else. After all, most doctors are not well trained in labor support, in breathing techniques and the like, as is the midwife.

"If there are any complications, if the patient is on a lot of drugs, the doctor becomes intensely occupied with her and the midwife stays on in a traditional nursing role. If another woman enters the hospital in labor, the doctor can stay with his ill patient while the midwife leaves the first patient and attends to the healthy newcomer. In a place where the contract is clear, the doctor feels no guilt, does a better job, and the patients are completely happy with the arrangement.

"In obstetrics," continues Dr. Franklin, "the doctor has tended to feel that his role is to look for the abnormal. This is what he is trained for and still wants to do. Today's increasing medical sophistication—amniocentesis, electronic fetal monitoring and the like—is increasing his abilities to pick up the abnormal. It has given the doctor more to learn, to master. It has tended to isolate him, make him more technically oriented and given him less time for the patient.

"On the other hand he needs to deal with the emotions aroused by pregnancy. Because he is the one whom the patient trusts with the total pregnancy.

"So we feel there's a need to bring a new person in —the nurse-midwife—to help fill some of these gaps.

"This doesn't mean that the nurse-midwife is looking after the emotional care of the mother, but the nurse-midwife makes the patient feel more secure around delivery. She does some of the normal examinations and then, if there are any deep emotional problems, allows the doctor time to sit and talk with the patient as much as necessary about these.

"While the nurse-midwife does not usually have a background in psychology or psychotherapy, she contributes much to the emotional needs of the patient. While she's taking care of routine things, she's saying, 'You're all right; you don't have to see the doctor today. I can handle it. That pain that you have in your side is related to the position of the baby. I am a competent person. I have enough knowledge to convince you that what I say is correct. I can furthermore prepare you for labor.

"And so the patient then comes to trust the midwife. When she goes into labor, she isn't confronted with a new woman she hasn't seen before. She sees someone she has come to believe in."

The roles that supernurses assume in Bellflower, Madison, and Philadelphia are not cast in cement. Other experiments in different parts of the country are made up of somewhat different combinations of responsibilities and talents, for the field is in a state of flux. Those who direct the Wisconsin and other programs concede that their supernurses could evolve into midwives, though not immediately because of legal restrictions, and the long, slow, expensive process of putting together a graduate training program in nurse-midwifery. Midwives, on the other hand, are being encouraged in many areas to broaden their scope to include such gynecological areas as contraception and cancer detection.

Dr. Franklin believes that the midwife is the chief solution to the expected manpower problem in the birth field. "My fear," he says, "is that the duties of the obstetrical nurse will just be expanded, that she will become the substitute for the missing first-year obstetrical resident. That her contract will be open-ended so that she is given duties for which she is not fitted or which don't always have a lot of gratification.

"The new supernurse might become a technologist, concerned with such things as monitoring, watching lines going up and down on a screen, with things that can be handled by a technician who doesn't need to have any social or personal skills.

"The nurse-midwife refuses to become a technologist. So I would prefer to have the midwife come back into the American care system rather than to place the emphasis on obstetrical nurses or paramedical people. The nurse-midwife was delivering babies before doctors were. She *belongs*. And my hope is that as more midwives become available, they will become more visible in training programs with obstetrical residents, who will learn to appreciate and work with them. This happens: Of requests for nurse-midwives that have come into New York's Maternity Center Association—from some forty institutions over a period of eighteen months—most originated with physicians who worked with nurse-midwives when they were residents or interns."

Will America in general accept nurse-midwives?

"There's been no trouble in getting the public to accept the nurse-midwife, wherever she's been tried," says Kitty Ernst. "Acceptance by the physician is the key. If physicians do not put wholehearted support behind nurse-midwifery, it's just going to struggle along as it has for the last forty years in this country. This is why it has struggled. It's as plain as the nose on your face.

"The question is: Is our commitment toward improving patient care or is our commitment toward improving doctor-patient care?"

In the view of patients and physicians who know them best, supernurses like Kitty Ernst and Rosalyn Powell are not second-best substitutes for busy M.D.s. Working in concert with doctors, these skilled professionals increase the quality of care.

CHAPTER

XV

Childbirth—Family Style

John, a middle-aged father, smiles ruefully as he recalls the birth of his daughter twenty years before in an exceptionally antiseptic hospital:

"I wasn't allowed to be with my wife during her labor and delivery. It was against the rules. I would get in the way, the nurses said, and I would contaminate my wife and baby and everything by bringing in my 'street germs.'

"Even after the birth, I wasn't supposed to see my wife. And so I would sneak up the fire escape every night, into her window, and visit with her while she ate a piece of chocolate cake or steak I'd brought her. Until one night the nurse caught us. She was horrified!"

In the name of progress, one generation accepts a situation that a previous generation would have considered ludicrous. John himself had been born at home, as was the prevailing custom all over America until about 1940. His father was at his mother's side throughout labor and delivery, holding her hand, comforting her, and even helping the doctor with the anesthesia. John's Aunt Lu was in and out of the bedroom; his grandmother was taking care of his brothers and sisters who played and waited just outside the door for the first sight of their new brother. In the kitchen, two neighbor women had arrived with casseroles and freshly baked pies. Birth then, as it had been for a million years and more, was very much a family affair.

"During the 1930s and '40s," explains University of Wisconsin neonatologist Stanley Graven, M.D., "we moved obstetrics, maternity care, and newborn care out of the home and into the hospital. From a warm and comforting atmosphere, surrounded by family and friends, the mother-to-be was suddenly transported into a barren hospital ward with only a nurse and her aide running back and forth to attend to thirty-two patients, with rules barring the father from the labor and delivery rooms, and more rules separating the new mother from her infant. Suddenly the mother and child were isolated.

"For too long we have failed to remember those things that went on in the home during childbirth that made adding a member to the family a tremendously exciting, great event. We put birth into a hospital where it sort of got sterilized, and where, in the process, a lot of the things we need most were lost. We have to go back and find these."

The search to renaturalize human birth is under way at hospitals large and small across America, most often under the banner of family-centered maternity care.

But why is it necessary? Almost all births are medically well-managed. Isn't that what really matters?

Why bother with fancy trimmings? "I've been work-ing in the maternity ward for twenty-five years," sniffs a veteran nurse, "and I don't know what the fuss is all about."

The fact is that scientific studies are at last confirm-ing something that many mothers have long felt—that the present traditional health-care system frequently is damaging to mothers, babies, and to the launching of new families. The damage begins before birth, in the form of increased nervous stress upon the mother; the stress causes a more difficult and potentially more dangerous birth. At birth and shortly thereafter, the system interferes with the crucial cementing of family ties—between mother and baby, mother and father, all three together. It interferes with breast-feeding, with resultant physical distress to both baby and mother. Finally, it may on some occasions cause last-ing emotional damage that contributes to emotional instability, child abuse, and the breakup of the family, troubles endemic in America today.

"Before a baby is born," says Dr. Stanley Graven, "it's a phantom, an unknown. The moment it's born, it's an *it*, a person you can see. The critical adjustment for a mother and father is to make that baby 'mine' and 'ours'—not a him or a her or an it that I own. This requires a very positive emotional output; you can't do it passively. And sometimes it happens that a baby goes home from the hospital as an object which the parents own but isn't part of them yet. Sometimes the final adjustment is never made; I can think of a case now—a mother with a child twelve or thirteen years old who's a 'him' but not a 'mine.' For a variety of reasons, the transition was never made."

Making birth natural once more isn't the simple thing it might seem. Says Dr. Graven: "You've got 'family-centered care' as a phrase that people in obstet-rics use. If you want a literal translation, they mean, 'Now that we have family-centered care, fathers can be in the labor room and maybe the delivery room, we let mothers come into the nursery and we let fathers put on a gown and hold their baby occasionally. We have some classes, too, in which Dad learns to diaper a baby, and we take the future parents on a hospital tour. And that constitutes family-centered care.' Be-cause that's really what's done differently.

"But this set of changes is just a little improvement over what we used to do. It's mostly just a veneer. Without really understanding why you do it. It's not really a deep change in philosophy and approach to childbirth.

"All right, you say, what really is family-centered childbirth, or what should it be? And I would refer you to investigators like Dr. Marshall Klaus, who has just returned from a year in Europe studying child-bearing in several cultures, and who has conducted some fascinating demonstrations of his own."

Neonatologist Marshall H. Klaus, M.D., is profes-sor of pediatrics and director of nurseries at Case Western Reserve University in Cleveland. As we talked in his study at University Hospital, the years slipped away and we were back in prehistory beside a flickering fire as a Cro-Magnon woman gave birth. For Marshall Klaus's thoughts have carried him far back into man's past, and into the animal kingdom, in a hunt for clues that will enable modern man to recon-struct the natural ecology of childbirth.

Human birth, believes Dr. Klaus, is part of a web of deep instinctual processes shaped by nature for man's optimum benefit. These instincts are still strong within the human mother, for they are based upon needs so fundamental that, had they not been met, the human race would never have survived.

There is first of all the need, Dr. Klaus explained, in the hours preceding birth, for privacy, peace, solitude, for a retreat from the possible harmful influences of the outside world.

Thus, as birth approaches, a mother cat finds a secret hiding place in which to give birth—under a porch, in a garage loft, deep in a haymow. A primitive human mother would have retreated to the place where she felt most safe—ideally, the family cave, protected by the clubs and spears of her husband and tribemates from the roving lynx and the saber-tooth tiger.

But what if the mother were far from home, in a strange place, perhaps among strangers when the birth pangs started?

Then her fear and uneasiness would have saved her and her young from birth in possibly dangerous surroundings. Her birth process would have been delayed for hours—long enough, perhaps, for her to retreat to the family cave.

How this works in animals was demonstrated by the team of Drs. Niles Anne Newton, Michael Newton, Donald Foshee, and Dudley Peeler. They frightened mice in labor—rather gently, simply by picking up a mother mouse after she gave birth to her first pup and holding her in cupped hands for one minute. The birth of the next pup did not occur until twenty minutes later, versus twelve minutes in the case of the undisturbed mother. (The human equivalent would be a delay of nearly two hours.) Even more striking was another experiment: a few hours before labor was expected, mother mice were placed in glass fishbowls containing the odor of cat urine. Their labors were delayed; it took four hours longer for them to give birth, the equivalent in humans of a delay of fifty-six hours.

In a stressful situation, nature delays labor at a price —of pain, and possible loss. Fear tightens the muscles and contracts the blood vessels of the mother's body. In an extreme situation, apparently this can so decrease the flow of life-giving blood to the fetus that it dies. Dr. Niles Anne Newton, a mother of four who is one of the nation's leading investigators into the psychology of childbirth, has shown that mother mice stressed during labor have more stillbirths.

It follows that human birth may also be more protracted, difficult, painful, and dangerous if the mother is fearful. More pain medication is necessary, with increased risk of side effects and interference with the natural birth and postbirth processes, including breast-feeding. More interference by the doctor may be necessary—more use of forceps, of Cesarean section.

Thus, family-centered care is not a kind of fancy fringe benefit proffered to pamper suburban mothers. Prenatal classes for mothers and fathers, and prenatal counseling increase a mother's knowledge and thereby decrease the fears that can cause trauma at time of birth. So does training in prepared or natural childbirth, whether or not the mother finally requires medication—at least she'll probably require *less*. There are scientific reasons to satisfy the ancient maternal desire for protection, security, warmth, and family support during childbirth, to as much as possible transfer the warm home setting into the hospital. There are scientific reasons *not* to separate the laboring woman from her husband and surround her with strangers, *not* to annoy her with noise and bustle, *not* to stress her with unnecessary procedures.

"Why do we subject human mothers to so much

environmental disturbance in labor?" asks Dr. Niles Anne Newton. "Why do we shave laboring women's pubic hair? Statistically, studies show no health advantage in this ritual shaving, which is humiliating and disturbing to women in labor. Why do we persist in moving a woman, as birth climax approaches, from the comfort of bed to a precipitous table in a strange new room in which she is expected to push her baby into space, hoping someone will catch it? Why not leave her comfortably in bed, back propped up in a simulated squatting position? Why do we ignore physiological needs in labor by the custom of placing women absolutely flat for delivery? Actual controlled studies have shown that the sitting position increases the woman's ability to push and that squatting alters the shape of the pelvic outlet in a way advantageous to labor."

"If you think about it," says Dr. Klaus, "there's something very abnormal about delivering in a hospital. The hospital changes everything. And it may not always be a change for the better."

A key interest of Dr. Klaus is the bond that must be established at birth between the mother and infant.

"You can see why the early mother-to-infant bond was so important thousands of years ago. There were wild animals about, perhaps attracted by the smell of blood from the birth and discarded membranes. The human infant cannot care for himself. He has to be picked up and held and put to the breast. There's no way he can approach his mother, as does the baby goat or lamb.

"He must be irresistible to his mother so she will pick him up and quickly form a tight bond with him; otherwise he'll be killed. He contributes to this attachment of bonds, this lovemaking, with his eyes.

"At birth, a normal baby who's had a normal deliv-

ery has brilliant eyes (before the silver nitrate ointment is put into them as a health measure). The baby's
eyes easily follow you—despite the fact that after that
first hour you cannot get him to follow easily for five
to six weeks; perhaps because after that first hour he
is overwhelmed by all other kinds of stimuli which
seem equally important."

Robin White, a youthful mother and writer-
researcher who has been helping the Klaus team test
the intelligence of newborns, confirms Klaus's observations: "These babies are so alert in the first half hour
or forty-five minutes! They're looking all around. And
if you hold them, they'll stare at you the whole time.
I can see how appealing a baby must be to his mother
if she gets him right after birth when he is so alert.
And why the eyes are so important. I can hear myself
saying, when I'm holding the baby, as he dozes off,
'Come on, open them, I want to see what your eyes
look like!' That's something I didn't have when my
own son was born. He's nine now. He was born at
nine in the morning and I didn't see him until the next
day."

"Dr. Niles Newton," says Dr. Klaus, "has made a
very important observation that there's a similarity
between intercourse, the birth of a baby, and breast-
feeding. For example, in all cases, the uterus contracts
rhythmically. One of the things you notice if you put
a nude baby next to the mother is a specific 'getting
acquainted' sequence shown in motion pictures we
have taken. First she begins to touch the infant's toes
and fingers and within eight minutes proceeds to mas-
saging his entire trunk, eventually exploring much of
the body. This might also be compared with the nuz-
zling and licking of her newborn by an animal
mother. It's an identification, examining process.

"However, in humans during this period there's

increasing eye-to-eye contact. And if you cover the eyes, the mother is upset. If the baby's eyes are closed because he's asleep, it will often be a day or two before the mother fully believes that the baby is hers.

"Another part of this is that, during this episode, the mother is excited. A physician who recently became a mother told me that, after her baby was born, she got very unusual feelings that she would *kill* a person who would at all harm the baby. That she would *die* for the baby. That was so atypical of her, and it was inappropriate to the situation, for no one was going to hurt her baby."

Yet this same urge would have proved most useful in primitive times, if wild animals were lurking around the birth site. As a boy growing up on a farm I'd repeatedly observed the ferocity of new animal mothers protecting their young. A normally placid cow was more dangerous than any mad bull, if her calf seemed in danger. A mother of piglets could be a menace.

Dr. Klaus is still seeking to determine whether or not there is a sensitive period after birth during which human bonding can be distorted. It has already been documented in animals, and varies among different species. In goats, sheep, and cattle, says Klaus, when a mother is separated from her young in the first hour or the first few hours after delivery and then the two are reunited, the mother will show disturbances of mothering behavior, such as butting her own off-spring away. But if mother and offspring stay together during the first four days and are separated on the fifth day, upon reunion the mother will recognize and claim her offspring as her own. During the critical first few days, a lasting bond has been formed.

"I would guess," says Dr. Klaus, "that in humans

the critical attachment time is also in the first week of life. Furthermore, the more contact the mother has with her baby, the sooner she touches it, holds it, fondles it, she may have less bleeding, she'll feel better, she'll be stronger. I believe there's a reciprocal action of the mother on the baby and the baby on the mother. This has not been scientifically demonstrated, but many people have written papers on it, and if a mother of a 'preemie' or ill baby goes into the nursery with her baby, she tends to move about much more easily and quickly. It is as if contact with the baby causes the release of maternal hormones which help her body return to normal."

In *Child and Family*, Drs. Niles and Michael Newton describe this reciprocal action as it occurs in completely natural breast-feeding: "The baby is put to the breast immediately after delivery. His sucking instinct is already fully developed so that he catches hold of the nipple and begins sucking. This sucking sets off the milk ejection reflex in the mother with the resultant discharge of oxytocin. Thus, the uterus is stimulated to contract vigorously. [Repeated contractions of the enlarged uterus in the weeks following birth enable it to expel fluids and shrink to its former small size.] The mother returns rapidly to a normal physical state so that she can devote her full energies toward her baby.

"Mother and baby stay close together after birth. Skin contact with the mother stimulates the baby's desire to nurse. Proximity to the baby increases the mother's interest in him. The baby is put to the breast whenever he indicates discomfort. This feeding act helps to warm and soothe him. He may stay at the breast for a half hour or an hour at a time. The comfort he receives there encourages him to fuss for frequent repetition. The hours of sucking each day vigorously stimulate lactation. Milk in large quantities appears rapidly, often within 24 hours after birth.

"The baby and mother stay near each other through the first few months. Each night they sleep within touching distance, and in the daytime the baby is carried everywhere his mother goes. Feeding continues on demand day and night. The baby seldom cries, for he is constantly within reach of the soothing comfort of his mother's breast, the warmness of her body, and the gentle touch of her skin.

"The mother in turn has an intense physical desire for her baby. She is under the influence of the hormone prolactin, which has been demonstrated to increase maternal behavior in other mammals. Furthermore, she needs the baby at regular intervals to empty her breasts, which otherwise become heavy and painful. Finally, each successful breastfeeding causes the uterus to contract, as it does at the time of female orgasm. The survival of the race for the millions of years before the concepts of 'conscience' and 'duty' were invented depended on the intense satisfaction gained from the acts of reproduction. Breastfeeding, like coitus, had to be pleasurable and satisfying if the race were to continue."

By contrast, a typical modern mother-baby scene is described by Mrs. Edwina Froehlich, executive secretary of the breast-feeding La Leche League: "The baby is crying in the nursery because he is away from his mother. His mother lies alone in her bed, uncomfortable because her breasts are engorging. Science enters the picture and tries to soothe the baby with a new nursery instrument that plays to the babies the amplified sound of a mother's heartbeat. Science treats the mother by giving her a pill to dry up her breasts. The baby gets a bottle of cow's milk.

"Neither problem would exist if mother and infant were permitted to snuggle up to each other as they did before the days of hospital deliveries when breast-feeding flourished."

Even breast-feeding under standard hospital conditions is usually a losing proposition. Dr. Niles Newton speaks of "token breastfeeding" as being the typical American pattern, "characterized by severe limitation of sucking by social customs from the day of birth to the day of eventual total weaning, which usually occurs within a few weeks. There are rules restricting the number of feedings, the duration of feedings, the amount of time between feedings, and the amount of mother-baby contact that stimulates the urge to suck."

Most U.S. hospitals, Mrs. Froehlich reports, are still unsupportive and unsympathetic to nursing mothers. So are most obstetricians and pediatricians "unless their own wives have breast-fed." Most doctors recommend supplemental feeding, which is unnecessary and destructive to the breast-feeding process.

The maternity nursing director of an Evergreen Park, Illinois, hospital tells how her hospital regulations read until recently: ". . . the baby was to be put to the breast one minute the first day, three minutes the second day, increasing to four or five minutes on the third day. The infants were taken out to their mothers only three times the second day."

Mother Nature would not approve.

In one of the decade's most striking experiments in human psychology, Dr. Klaus and an associate, John H. Kennell, M.D., have shown that apparently they can alter mothers' behavior simply by adding a few extra hours of close contact between mother and baby during the first few days of life.

Two groups of fourteen women each, randomly

chosen, from similar backgrounds, were allowed to see their babies for a short time right after birth, again briefly six to twelve hours later, and for twenty to thirty minutes every four hours for bottle feedings. All, in short, were given the standard American hospital treatment for mothers and newborns.

However, the first group in addition was provided an extra sixteen hours of close baby-mother contact during the first three to four days of the baby's life.

In this group, during the first two or three hours after birth, the mother was given an added hour with the baby nude in her bed.

Then, for the next three days only, the mother had the baby, but not nude, for an extra five hours, perhaps from 1 to 6 P.M.

("We brought the baby into the mother's room in a bassinet," says Dr. Klaus, "but to our surprise the mother would usually take him out of the bassinet and into the bed with her.")

That was all. Otherwise the two groups were treated exactly the same. But differences in mothering behavior between the two groups were noticed immediately, and continued.

After one month, mothers in the first group were more likely to pick up their babies when they cried, were more reluctant to leave their babies, and thought about them more when they did. During a physical examination at the pediatrician's office, they were more likely to soothe their infants and stay by their sides.

When the babies were thirty days old, a fifteen-minute feeding was filmed through one-way glass by a time-lapse movie camera operating at one frame per second. Each of the first six hundred frames was scored by analyzers looking for one or more of twenty-five specific activities, ranging from caretaking (such as proper bottle position) to eye-to-eye contact to cuddling and fondling. And again the first group of women got far higher mothering scores.

In further studies at age one year, the two groups were still different, during a stressed office visit.

"It's our impression," says Marshall Klaus, "that massive alterations in hospital procedures will be indicated once the behavioral requirements of mothers are determined. Under present practice, most normal deliveries in this country are associated with several days of deprivation for the mother."

What *should* happen after birth in the hospital of the future?

"Within twenty minutes after birth, after baby and mother are checked for their well-being, the baby is warmed and dried, and the placenta is delivered, we would put the mother and baby skin to skin and just leave them alone. We're trying to institute this procedure now with all of our full-term mothers, a time after delivery when the mother and baby have a period of privacy. In other words, you don't make love to your wife on a streetcar. It's a private affair. The attachment of bonds, which occurs in lovemaking, takes place best in privacy. We think the husband should also be there because this will bind the marriage much more tightly. We believe there's a crucial period in which the mother and the baby and the father should be together, without anybody around, with the baby nude as maximal stimulus.

"No eye ointment, I hope; that can wait until after the reunion; it can make the baby's eyes puffy, and if the baby's eyes are shut the mother has difficulty in getting to know her baby.

"You have to use this first period when the baby's eyes are open—he can see his mother's face, you know, in the first hour. Then the mother becomes attached to the baby, and very possessive.

"In the days following birth, most mothers will have their babies with them at least six extra hours a day, in addition to the present feeding times. And I would think that the whole family, including the baby's brothers and sisters, should participate in getting acquainted with the baby in the hospital. You know, a standard maternity department is a rather depressing place for the mother, because the whole family isn't around. We should think about opening it up so the other children can come up, as they do in hospitals in Europe and throughout New Zealand. The risk of increased infection is not really significant, despite this excuse always given by hospitals for barring children.

"Another important change will come when we start thinking of the mother and the baby as a unit. Sometimes the baby is ready to go home but the mother doesn't really know how to take care of him yet. So she should stay in the hospital until she feels relaxed and confident in handling him.

"That's another advantage of 'extended visiting' by the baby, as we call it. [Rooming in.] The mother learns how to care for her baby. She knows what a sneeze and a cough and the cries mean before she goes home with the baby.

"In Holland, where I was visiting, they wait until the mother can complete the baby's bath. She almost has a test that must be passed before she can leave the hospital."

Babies and parents in special circumstances would also be treated differently in the ideal hospital of the future, says Dr. Klaus:

"We think you have to reevaluate the whole system —not only for the benefit of the mother and the normal baby, but for the mother of the premature baby, the mother of the ill, malformed, dying, or stillborn baby, and for the mother who adopts.

"The mother of the premature baby, immediately after delivery, may on occasion be able to have her baby fairly close to her. She'll be able to go into the intensive-care nursery and touch and even help care for her baby. We may find a way to let preemies go home sooner than they now do. Several studies have made the shocking discovery that twenty-five to forty percent of battered children in this country originally were patients in a premature nursery. Versus six percent of the population in general. And I think this situation was *produced* in part because we haven't made a place for the family or the mother in the care of preemies.

"If the mother of a preemie has not had good mothering herself, didn't want the baby, if she's especially young and unmarried, doesn't have a good home to go to, if in the hospital she doesn't get to see the baby for two to three weeks, or sees it only through glass, it's not going to be easy for her to develop a close bond with the infant.

"Another very important element also operates here. We bring in a lot of ill babies from other hospitals to our intensive-care nursery. But once we do this, the mother believes her baby is going to die. Even if *we* know it's not going to. And so we try to do everything we can to prevent this premature mourning.

"Let me give you an example. If I told you Jack Kennedy were alive, you wouldn't believe it. Because you, and the whole nation, have mourned his loss. So if for one day the mother has mourned that her baby may die, it's very hard for her to turn around immediately and take her baby home, to accept him.

"So what we do routinely is to use the father as liaison between the mother and baby. We have him come from the original hospital to ours in his own car. He stays two to four hours with us, comes into the nursery, drinks coffee with us, takes a Polaroid picture of the baby to show to his wife. Then he goes back and reports to his wife.

"If we don't do something like this, the father goes into a great panic. We've noticed in cases of ill babies that the father tends to be hyperactive, to start going around rather aimlessly from place to place, and the mother tends to be very quiet. We try to mobilize the father's activity for some useful purposes, such as communicating with his wife, coming in every day for a couple of hours, helping care for his baby, being both a father and a mother to it."

There is much frontier remaining for Dr. Klaus and his team to explore. For example, they are trying to discover whether better mothering (induced by better bonding) results in smarter children. And whether adoptive parents should receive their new baby immediately after delivery, instead of three to six weeks later.

One obstetrician who follows the investigations of Drs. Klaus and Kennell very carefully is Booth Maternity Center Chief, Dr. John Franklin, a member of the committee on family-centered maternity care of the American College of Obstetricians and Gynecologists.

"I think," he says, "that the Klaus concept of maternal attachment should be taught in obstetrics as thoroughly as is pelvimetry. The fact is that you can always do a Cesarean section, almost always get the baby out in time in an emergency. A far greater need is to help prevent the problems people have today in childrearing.

"The sociologists have delineated the forces that are focused in upon the nuclear family—two parents and a child, bereft of supporting relatives, old neighbors, and good friends. And these forces result in destruction a third of the time, or more, with the divorce of the parents, with the child suffering. So that the behavioral aspects of obstetrics and family life are now accounting for a good bit of sickness.

"Probably a good many illnesses are somatic expressions of emotional problems resulting from the sick marriage and the sick family. To me, it's as much of a problem as a high-risk pregnancy.

"I think doctors are beginning to know what family-centered care is because their patients are demanding it. Patient-education groups like ASPO, the American Society for Psycho-Prophylaxis in Obstetrics (Lamaze method); the Childbirth Education Association; and La Leche League are quite consistent about what they want: fathers in the delivery room, close ties between the mother and child, not much medication, support for prepared or natural childbirth and for breast-feeding.

"I think attachment behavior such as Klaus has described gives the doctor a new agenda. And that is to see if the patient is accepting her pregnancy, her role as a mother-to-be, and then, after she delivers, to see whether she's accepting her child.

"Ideally, family-centered maternity care begins with the first visit to the obstetrician. By the husband as well as the wife. Here at Booth we encourage husbands to come at every visit, and we schedule office visits on evenings and Saturdays to make this possible.

"We feel that the husband has the same task as the

wife does. That he accept the fact that his wife is pregnant. That he accept the fact that he's going to be a father and to like the kid. He's working on these same three points in a slightly different way, and we try to get both future parents to talk about their feelings.

"At that first visit we discuss the expectations of the parents. And by raising these questions, the obstetrician has approved and set in motion their working on it. But if the obstetrician says, 'I've examined you and your bones and hemoglobin are thus and so, and you're okay.' And if he says nothing about the feelings of pregnancy, then the patient will get the same message she probably got at home: 'I want you to be a good kid and I don't want to hear about your feelings.'

"And she and her husband will rear their child in the same way. They will attempt to toilet-train and socialize him as fast as possible, will try to have him do as well as possible in school without objecting to the irrationalities of the schools. They won't permit discussion of the irrationalities of the home, or the arbitrariness of the rules, and they won't permit the child to grow. The way to permit a child to grow is to say, 'Hey, he can't help his feelings, let's try to understand why he feels the way he does.' And that begins at birth."

Booth Maternity Center provides a pure example of family-centered maternity care. Its differences from the standard American hospital start with the way it is organized, which reflects its responsiveness to the families it serves. Although final authority for planning and policy rests with the sponsoring organization, the Salvation Army, all decisions affecting patient care are arrived at in consensus with a consumer board including recent mothers and mothers-to-be, among them unwed teen-agers.

Midwives conduct most prenatal examinations, lead prenatal classes in husband-coached prepared childbirth, and stay with each patient continuously during labor and delivery.

All paper work is done beforehand so there is no annoying delay at the desk at the time of admission.

The laboring mother is free to move about the hospital, rather than being confined to bed. Her husband or other support person may be with her throughout labor and delivery.

"The fact is," says midwife Kitty Ernst, "within the limits of safety the mother's wishes are held paramount. For example, if everything's going well and the mother has a real desire to avoid the delivery table and deliver in her labor bed, we respect her wishes.

"We may say to her in labor, 'You seem to have a little difficulty relaxing. The contractions seem rather bothersome. How do you feel about it?'

"And she may say, 'I'm doing fine.' And so we don't administer a pain-killing drug, unless she asks us to. We don't shave the pubic hair, nor give an enema, nor do an episiotomy routinely. We don't strap a woman to the delivery table.

"By getting the mother to participate in childbearing decisions, we help her build confidence in herself and her ability to do things—which I think is essential for motherhood. If you're going to raise children, you should start with a confidence base. We try to reinforce this rather than fragment it or break it down."

Immediately after delivery, mother and father are left alone for an extended period to touch and hold their baby. In the days following, the baby can stay in the same room with the mother continuously or be watched part of the time in a central nursery, as the mother wishes. There is a quiet room for breast-feeding mothers, and a day room where brothers and sisters of newborns can visit their mothers. Fathers are not considered visitors. They are not bound by rigid visiting hours, nor are there any restrictions about them being with the mother and handling the baby.

The entire atmosphere of Booth is an antidote to bad experiences that some of the mothers have had in other hospitals. Improper care, not family centered, can literally frighten a woman out of having another child. "We've had numerous patients," says Kitty Ernst, "who were absolutely petrified because they were pregnant again and because they feel that their previous experiences were nightmares."

"At Booth," says one new mother, "they treat you as if you were healthy, and that pregnancy is a healthy experience, not a disease."

"I think my husband and I were a flop in natural childbirth," says another. "I got plenty of drugs. But at home, before I went to the hospital, the training in breathing helped me. And knowing what would come next. That was the blessing—you knew what would come next, and so you wouldn't panic. And at Booth they gave my husband a role so he was comfortable."

"At Booth," says a young father, a teacher of high-school English, "I was allowed to become involved in the birth and not feel like a helpless outsider. I had long wondered at the stereotyped portrait of the man who takes his wife to the hospital and then leaves her, goes to a bar and drinks himself silly and then comes back to the hospital hours later and sees his child through the nursery glass. Then sees his wife who says that everything is fine. I know now why that man had been drinking so much. It was because he knew that something was going on in which he was very much involved, something painful, but it was out of his hands and there was nothing he could do about it.

Almost everything he cared about was suddenly at stake and so what could he do but drink?"

"During delivery," says a pretty nurse who came to Booth for the birth of her fourth child, "the object is to give the girl the chance to deliver the baby slowly, to push it out, rather than to have the doctor deliver the baby.

"The people here were marvelous," she continues. "And my husband was with me the whole time, helping to coach me in my breathing. As soon as our baby was born, the midwife put him up on my abdomen so my husband and I could touch him, then they cut the cord, and in a few minutes my husband and I and the baby were alone together, getting acquainted.

"I had only a little medication, which didn't affect the baby. And he was so alert. I think he responded to my touch, because he sort of quieted down as soon as I picked him up from his warming cradle. When I offered him a breast, he went right to it; and as he nursed, the uterus contracted so strongly I could feel it squeezing out the blood. I was filled with such a marvelous maternal feeling.

"I think my first reaction after the birth of my baby was love to my husband. Because we had shared such a marvelous moment. And that he was such a help to me. And then after that came love to the baby. We had a little bit of time there to share feelings with each other. And I wanted to just look at him. I wanted just to stare at him and hug him and hold him—my husband, that is. And then after that it was as if I drew strength from my husband to go ahead and take care of the baby with the love from both of us. It was very beautiful. And my husband said, 'Gee, I wish we could go back and do our other births over again."

Dr. Franklin is not sure that the Booth kind of atmosphere can be duplicated in the superhospitals of the future.

"My concern," he says, "is that there is enormous economic pressure to centralize deliveries to a minimum volume of two thousand deliveries a year. This is a trend the American College of Obstetricians and Gynecologists has supported; it is the only way for an obstetric service to be economically viable. And my fear is that this will lead to increasing regimentation of patients.

"If the nurse-midwife is used in a large service like this, and if the doctors will accept any part of family-centered care, there is still hope that the patients will find an individual expression in this system.

"But I'm afraid that there will be elaborate rules about the baby rooming in with the mother, about breast-feeding, about everything. These rules will have nothing to do with the natural needs of the baby, but instead with the convenience of the hospital staff."

In Wilmington, Delaware, there is proof that family-centered care can be a roaring success even in a large hospital. It's been so successful that the Wilmington General Division of Wilmington Medical Center, with five-thousand deliveries a year, has almost all of the baby business in town; two other maternity wards in town have closed down.

Mrs. Edith Wonnell, R.N., C.N.M., is coordinator of the Parent Education Department for the hospital, which was built in 1965 and consciously patterned after St. Mary's Hospital in Evansville, Indiana, the mother hospital of family-centered maternity care. Here, babies room in with their mothers for as many hours as their mothers wish.

Mrs. Wonnell directs a large program. At any time, there are ten groups of Preparation for Childbirth classes for expectant couples and four groups for clinic mothers going on simultaneously. Five nurse-instructors teach new mothers during their postpartum stay in the hospital. New mothers even have their choice of breast-feeding, child-care, family-adjustments, and infant-safety programs shown in their rooms via closed-circuit TV.

"At first," she says, "childbirth education emphasized only labor and delivery. Some childbirth education classes still confine themselves to this. Now we're going farther along in the process, by helping parents meet the new demands of parenthood."

One example of the gamut of supportive resources available at Wilmington is a Family Centered Parents group, which sponsors monthly seminars for new parents on such matters as toys, infant development, and teaching baby to talk.

A committee of nursing mothers has helped to raise the percentage of breast-feeding mothers at the hospital from 15 percent to more than 45 percent. At any one time, the committee consists of some thirty mothers, experienced in breast-feeding, who counsel up to three hundred expectant and nursing mothers on a one-to-one basis.

The entire program of parent education is self-supporting, mostly from prenatal class fees. There are donations, too, and fund-raising efforts by the parents' group. There is in addition a grant from state mental health funds.

"The state," says Mrs. Wonnell, "realizes that if we can get in on the ground floor, before a family starts to have trouble, we can prevent much mental illness from developing."

Dr. Marshall Klaus speaks of starting even earlier— twenty years earlier.

"Do you have a daughter? You know how she carries her dolls about, sings to them, tucks them into bed at night. She is really very loving with her dolls. As she will be with her own babies. She isn't just playing, she is rehearsing.

"They tell me that there are some films in New York showing mothers mothering their own little girls. And there are films of these same little girls twenty years later and they're mothering in the same way. In one sequence, a mother wipes off a playground slide, her two-year-old slides down, and then the mother grabs the child in her arms and hugs her. Time after time. This is followed by a series in which the two-year-old, now grown, follows exactly the same sequence with her daughter.

"If your daughter is going to be a mother, one of the most important things is that she see not only her mother as a model, but that she see other women as models—as happened a hundred or a thousand years ago when all the relatives lived together and there was always a new baby in the house or next door.

"So in schooling, preparation for life, children should have practical experience. And I don't mean just baby-sitting. When I was in Denmark I saw thirteen- and fourteen-year-old girls in the midwifery clinic helping with deliveries and with baby care. Why shouldn't teen-agers in this country work in hospitals caring for mothers and babies, perhaps later assist at a nursery school? They need to learn about taking care of the families they will have someday."

Mothering and fathering may be instinctual. But as each change in our world further rips the ancient web of human life, love and instinct need a bit more help.

The childbearing revolution involves much more than drastic changes in obstetrical practice. It requires an enlarged view of the human family and childbirth within it, not only by medical people but also by parents-to-be. The expressed wishes of tomorrow's parents can and will effect reform in the way new people are nurtured and brought into the world. A mother-to-be is not meant to be a passive recipient of care. She and her husband are Adam and Eve, central figures in the miraculous creation of a new life.

Index